The Alchemy Cookbook

Transforming Food into Medicine

Nicole Azzopardi

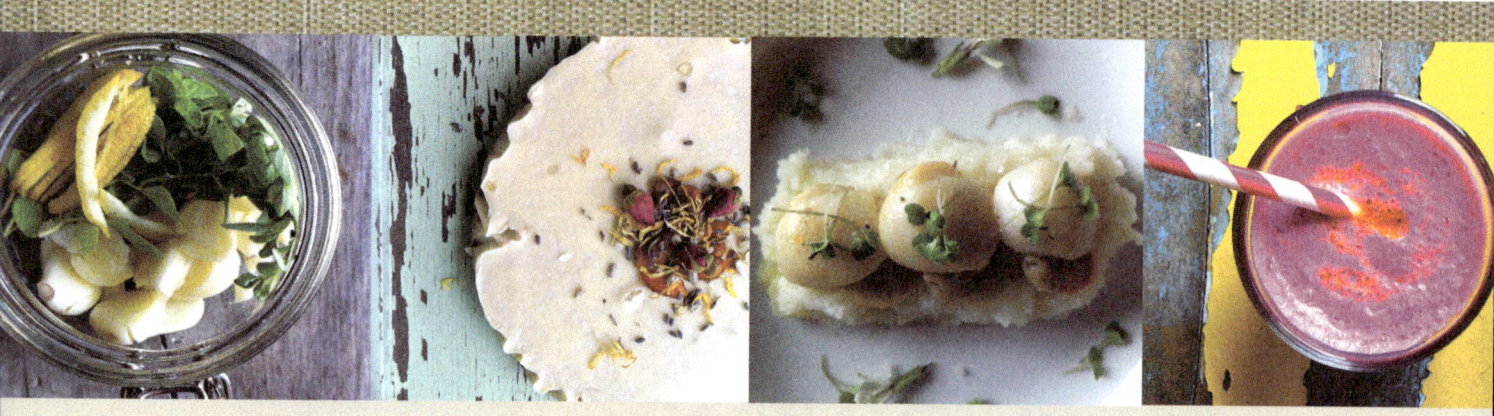

Disclaimer and Copyright Information

All information provided within this publication is for informational purposes only, and is not to be construed as medical advice or instruction. Please consult your physician or a qualified health professional on any matters regarding your health and wellbeing or on any opinions expressed within this publication. The information provided in this publication is believed to be accurate based on the best judgment of the author. However, you as the reader must be responsible for consulting with your own health professional on matters raised within. I, the author of The Alchemy Cookbook, will not accept responsibility for the actions or consequential results of any action taken by any reader.

The material in this guide may include information, products or services by third parties. Third Party Materials comprise of the products and opinions expressed by their owners. As such, I do not assume responsibility or liability for any Third Party material or opinions. The publication of such Third Party Materials does not constitute my guarantee of any information, instruction, opinion, products or services contained within the Third Party Material. Publication of such Third Party Material is simply a recommendation and an expression of my own opinion of that material.

No part of this publication shall be reproduced, transmitted, or sold in whole or in part in any form, without the prior written consent of the author. All trademarks and registered trademarks appearing in this guide are the property of their respective owners.

These statements have not been evaluated by the Therapeutic Goods Administration Code or Act. Any products discussed are not intended to diagnose, treat, cure, or prevent any disease. Users of this guide are advised to do their own due diligence when it comes to making decisions and all information, products and services that have been provided should be independently verified by your own qualified professionals.

Please be mindful of copyright - The Alchemy Cookbook is intellectual property that is protected by copyright law. It may not be republished or distributed, either for financial gain or not, without written permission of the author, Nicole Azzopardi. Contact Nicole at www.thealchemyprotocol.com with inquiries.

© Nicole Azzopardi. All Rights Reserved.

Design: Jackie Jackson Design.

Photography: Nicole Azzopardi.

www.thealchemyprotocol.com

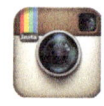

Mumma Care

The Alchemy Cookbook is Nicole Azzopardi's love letter to her children.

After searching for the most nutrient dense, healing food she could find to help heal her eldest daughter's damaged digestive system, Nicole found the very best medicine came from rediscovering some of our oldest traditions.

Simple, elegant and beautiful, the practice of culturing vegetables, making stocks and hearty soups and stews has provided the restorative qualities she had searched for.

Nicole's parents were born in Egypt. Her mother is Maltese/French and her father is Maltese/Greek.

She draws on the forgotten traditions of all of these cultures and more to create a delicious array of every day foods that heal.

> Foods that are quick and easy to make as well as foods the whole family can enjoy.

Her blog, Facebook and Instagram pages, Mumma Care, supports mothers and their children who are food allergic, intolerant and/or have autism. Nicole also teaches cooking classes and runs retreats on Victoria's Bellarine Peninsula.

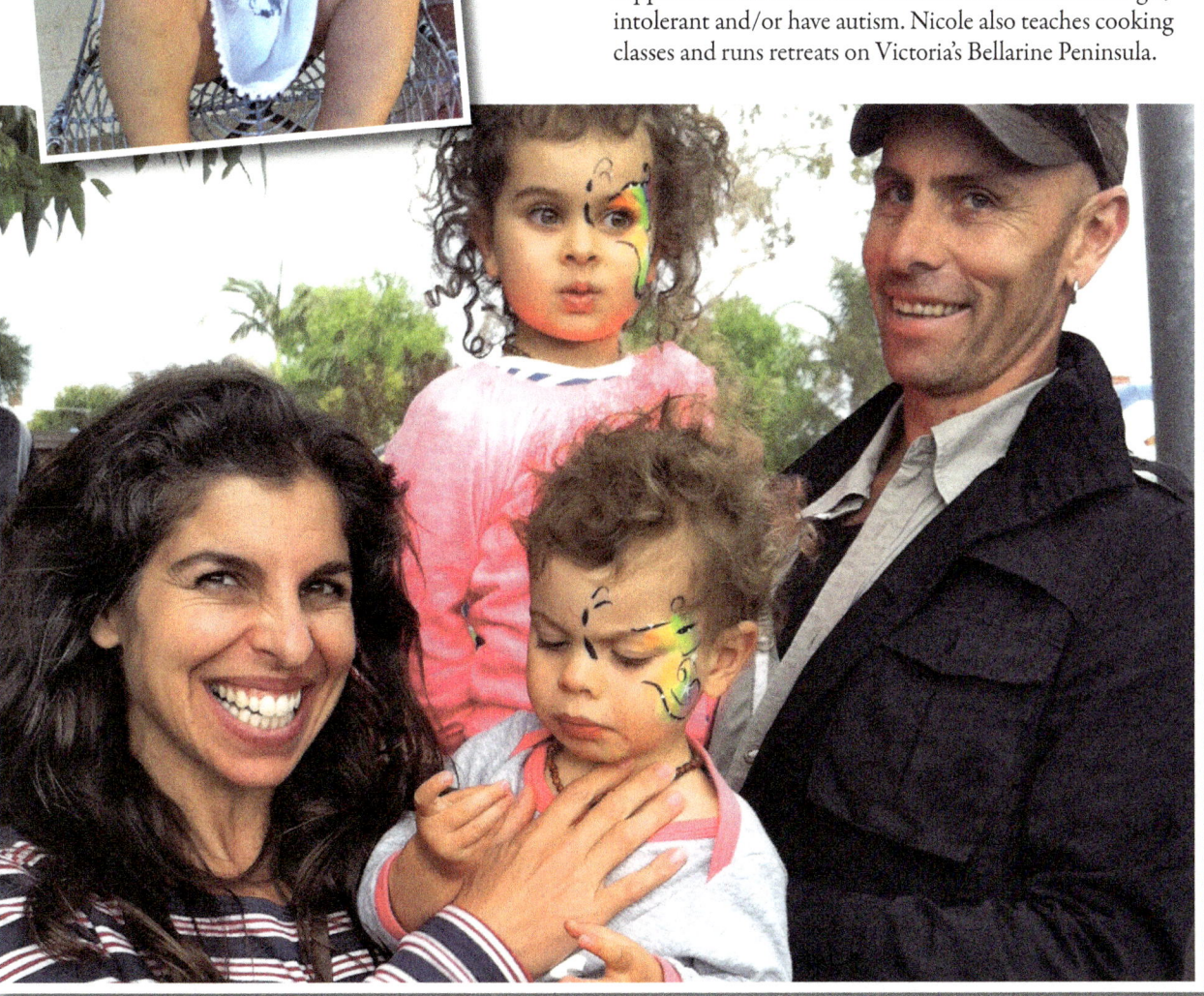

Contents

Mumma Care	3
Contents	4
For Stevie & Josie	5
The Alchemy Cookbook	6
Foreword and thanks	7
Our Story	8
Your Kitchen Apothecary	9

Getting started — 10

The Basics — 11
Cultured cream	12
Yoghurt	13
The mighty chicken stock	14

Condiments — 16

Salts — 18

Vanilla orange rind extract — 20

Culinary Probiotics — 21

Fermented foods — 22
Sauerkraut	24
Fermented garlic	26
Radish with kaffir lime leaves	28
Dilly sliced cucumbers	29
Middle Eastern beetroot & turnip mezze	30
Carrots sticks with mustard seeds & garden herbs	32
Spanish onion with thyme & garlic	34
Fermented beetroot with turmeric, orange rind & cinnamon	36
Dilly beans	38
Kimchi	40
Lacto fermented tomato salsa	42

Sides & Snacks — 43
Chicken liver pate	44
Slow roasted brussels sprouts with butter & rosemary	46
Gut healing jelly cups	48
Poached egg on salmon	50
Spiced beetroot carpaccio	52
Fried mushrooms with thyme	54

Soups — 55
Borscht	56
The easiest pumpkin soup ever	58
Cauliflower & leek soup	60
Greek-style chicken soup	62
Carrot, cabbage, marjoram & chicken soup	64

Main Meals — 67
Cauliflower mashed 'faux'tatoes, scallops & rocket micro greens.	68
Classic Sunday roast, buttered carrots, sage & rosemary salt	70
French-style pickled sardines with kimchi & lime	72
Sumac salted roast pork belly with sage carrots	74
Fish with radish & fennel	76
Honeyed roast chicken with tarragon, turnips, garlic & peas	78
Roasted swede stacks	80
Chicken casserole with herb 'pesto'	82
Greek style lamb cutlets, home made yoghurt with home grown mint, sauerkraut & pumpkin chips	84
That classic combination – fish & chips by the beach.	86
Scallops, cultured cream & herbs	88

Sweets for My Sweet — 89
Apple, orange, macadamia & date crumble	90
Turkish ginger & apricot cake	92
Date & rosewater melting moments	94
Instant chocolate raspberry ice cream	96
Mixed berry mousse	98
Raw honey panna cotta with vanilla & orange extract	100
Poached pears in turmeric & ginger	102
Gluten & grain free cookies	104
Two-minute cultured raspberry ice cream	105
Egyptian rosewater honey cake	106
Orange blossom blueberry pie	108
Banana cream brekky custards	110
Tropical coconut, mango, passionfruit creams	112
Blueberry jelly	114

Drinks — 115
Summer cocktails	116
Beetroot kvass: A deeply cleansing tonic.	118
Watermelon, young coconut, lemon & lime frappe	120
Green smoothies Vs Pink smoothies – which one is right for you?	122
Smoothies	123
The real deal: Probiotic mango avocado lassi.	124

For our friends with severe allergies. — 125

Afterword — 126

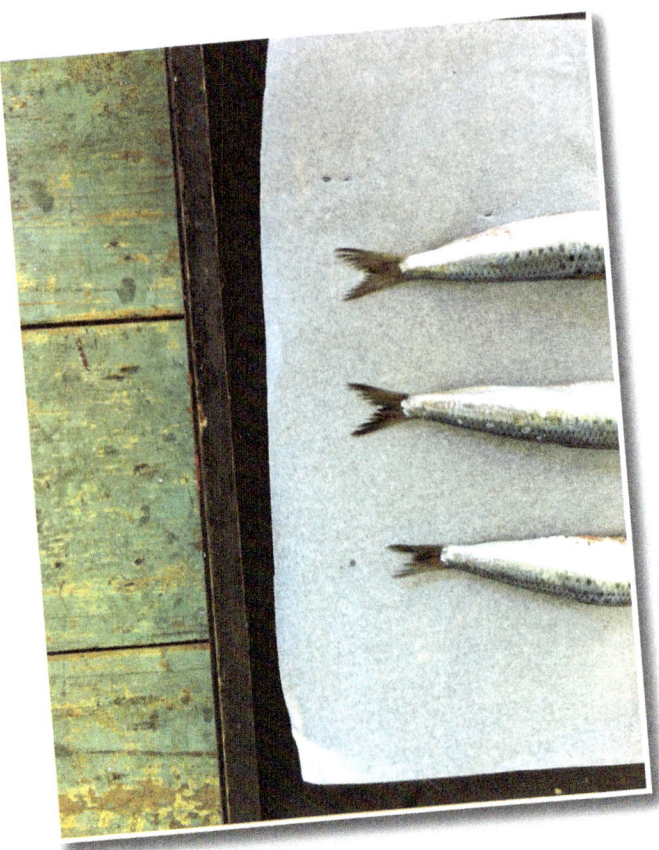

For Stevie and Josie

Everywhere I look
I see beauty.

My darling daughters, your sensitive tummies have forced me to open my eyes and look for solutions.

Turns out the answers are all around us - growing in technicolour.

I would have missed it all had it not been for you.

Forcing me into our garden and kitchen. Driving me to my books. Going back to the future to live in a way that suits your sensitive souls.

Away from the supermarket shelves, the boxes, the packets.

Learning, researching, cooking, eating, loving you both so much - your allergies have been your genius and your blessing to your father and I.

Every day we discover more of nature's secrets. They are beyond my wildest dreams.

Thank you.

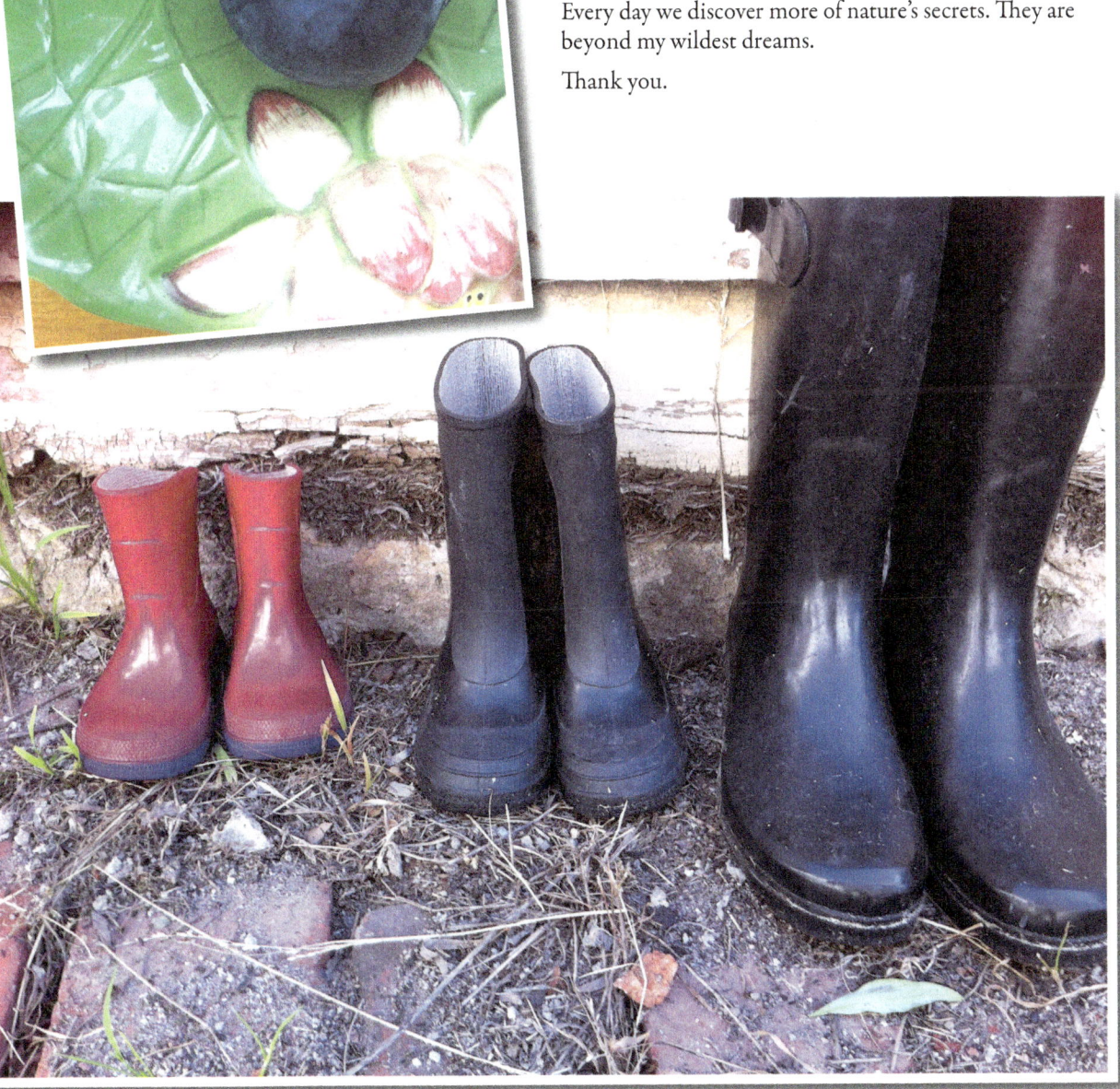

The Alchemy Cookbook

Transforming Food Into Medicine

Reviving the lost art of making culinary probiotics, The Alchemy Cookbook offers fresh, simple food for families that nourish, satisfy, detox & heal.

Join Nicole and her family for an international tour through the world of fermented foods, as well as taking a look at some exotic and delicious gluten, grain and sugar free desserts.

With recipes like Middle Eastern beetroot and turnip mezze, Turkish apricot cake and Egyptian pink lemonade, The Alchemy Cookbook is an example of how old-school traditions can become delicious solutions to many modern-day health dilemmas.

"One of the biggest barriers to the GAPS Diet initially was that I felt it was very egg and nut heavy," Nicole says.

"Stevie Rose was anaphylactic to these foods at the time and her histamine sensitivity excluded us from ferments and broths so I spent a lot of time learning about the diet but wondering how I could find our way in.

On various forums I kept reading accounts of people dropping their severe allergies. The thought of being able to lose the epipens forever was a freedom I really wanted to give our daughter if possible. The principles seemed sensible and we had nothing to lose by trying.

Within a few months of being on GAPS without eggs or nuts, allergy tests with our most excellent paediatric allergist Dr Peter Goss revealed that slowly but surely, all of Stevie's severe allergies were leaving her."

> Within six months of the diet, Stevie Rose no longer needed epipens. First it was the sesame that went, then all nuts - except peanuts - then eggs.

"I cannot explain this phenomenon," Nicole admits. "I don't believe anybody can at this point. Everyone is bamboozled by severe allergy and is working hard to find suitable answers. It is often explained that children outgrow their allergies, but what does outgrow mean? Can we lend a hand in the maturing and strengthening process - and even possibly accelerate it?

Like me, our allergist suspects that gut bacteria has a lot to do with it.

I wondered, if a lot of the body's immune system is found in the gut wall, then would it follow that if you strengthened the gut and fed it targeted healing foods, you would strengthen the immune system?

An immune system that is not under stress might not then react incorrectly towards harmless foods.

In addition, not having to deal with a massive amount of inflammation caused by gut distress, the immune system could then get on with its day to day tasks.

The GAPS Diet is not suitable for everyone but it has been life-changing for us.

I recommend any substitution of food groups be handled in conjunction with a trained professional.

The Alchemy Cookbook hopes to provide nourishing, healing alternatives for those living with restrictions or doing alternative diets."

Many of these recipes can easily be substituted.

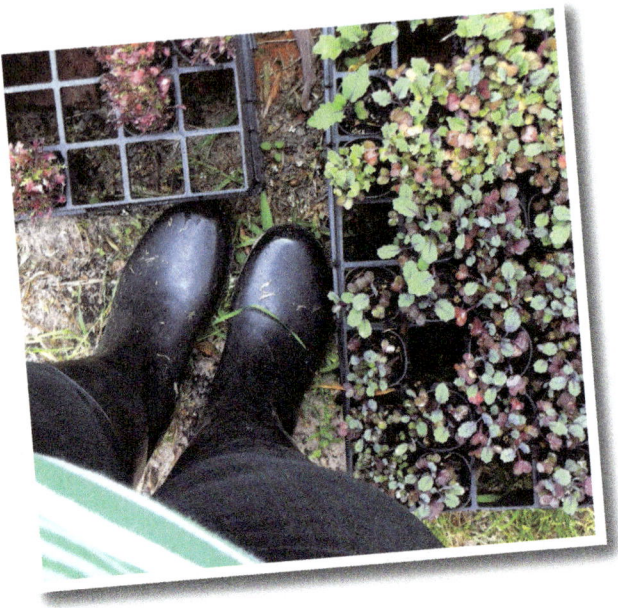

Foreword and thanks

To all the Facebook mums who are online sharing their inspiring stories of healing and recovery I thank you. Together we have shared our learnings, our recipes, our fears, our worries and our loneliness. Thank you for your encouragement and your international taste testing efforts!

Thank you to Dr Natasha Campbell-McBride, Marieke Rodenstein, Kitsa Yanniotis, Katerina Cosgrove and Bridie Williams.

Thank you to all the mums in our village who have gone out of their way to include us and understand the health challenges.

Books I love

Nourishing Traditions by Sally Fallon

Wild Fermentation by Sandor Katz

Wholefood for Children by Jude Blereau

Gut and Psychology Syndrome by Dr Natasha Campbell-McBride

Breaking the Vicious Cycle by Elaine Gottschall

Cultured Food for Life by Donna Schwenk

Healing with Whole Foods by Paul Pitchford

Herbal Antibiotics by Stephen Harrod Buhner

Ignite Your Spirit by Shakti Durga

Shonishin by Thomas Wernicke

Healthy Every Day by Pete Evans

Little French Kitchen by Rachel Khoo

Limoncello and Linen Water by Tessa Kiros

Saraban by Lucy and David Malouf

Colour of Maroc by Rob and Sophia Palmer

Stephanie Alexander's Kitchen Garden Companion

Grow Harvest Cook by Meredith Kirton and Mandy Sinclair

Thank you Ruth, Megan and Queenscliff Kindergarten for embracing a whole new way to explore food. It's been wonderful learning together.

Thank you Jackie for this most beautiful design work. You have done this from your heart and for the many children out there who may be helped from this story.

Thank you to my family. Greg Franzke, for helping to bring this project home, and special thanks to my mother, Ophelia.

"I would like to thank Nicole Azzopardi for this book! Wonderful recipes and explained in a way which makes them easy and simple to implement! I am sure that this book will become an essential companion to the families who are trying to heal their children and adults recovering from chronic illness around the world.

And what an inspiring story Nicole has to tell! She has demonstrated that allergies of any type are curable and no child or adult has to live with them for the rest of their lives! Her little girls are beautiful and it is great to see them involved with food! I am sure that all the hard work their mother has put into feeding them will allow them to grow up having a normal healthy relationship with food, which is so fundamental to the child's development. I am also sure that when Nicole's daughters have grown up they will become great cooks and will create healthy families of their own.

This book was written with great love and care! I warmly recommend it."

Dr Natasha Campbell-McBride, MD,
Author of *The Gut and Psychology Syndrome*

Our Story

The Alchemy Cookbook has come about because until recently our little girl was anaphylactic and intolerant to many foods.

As she grew older those foods irritated her gut and in turn affected her mind. From a newborn baby, she could not sleep, was colicky and had poor digestion.

As she grew, she began to bang her head, was terrified of household appliances, could not stand the feeling of a seat belt on her skin and would scream all day and through the night.

We tried everything to help her but finally realised that by working to heal and seal her gut wall with specific foods like meat stock and cultured vegetables, her symptoms slowly began to disappear.

I am delighted to say that our beautiful little girl is doing very well. She is calm and happy, she can eat many, many more foods and her favourites are avocado, cream and butter.

With gratitude and thanks I credit neurologist and nutritionist Dr Natasha Campbell-McBride and her book *Gut and Psychology Syndrome* with much of the healing that has occurred in our daughter Stevie Rose. It was this doctor who helped me to see the connection between the gut and the brain and how we could very effectively take healing into our own hands.

For more information about the GAPS Diet, please visit www.gaps.me

> Being a mother is a massive task. The Alchemy Cookbook is for any mother, new or experienced, looking for support.

Whether you are interested in learning how to do a bit more healthy eating, exhausted and drawing on reserves, can't work out why your newborn won't sleep, or overwhelmed by the responsibility of a child with anaphylaxis, food allergies or autism, this book hopes to provide you with a range of alternative wholefood staples that are allergy conscious, delicious and nutritious.

Let's begin today by delving into the world of gluten, grain and sugar free recipes and making your own delicious probiotic food.

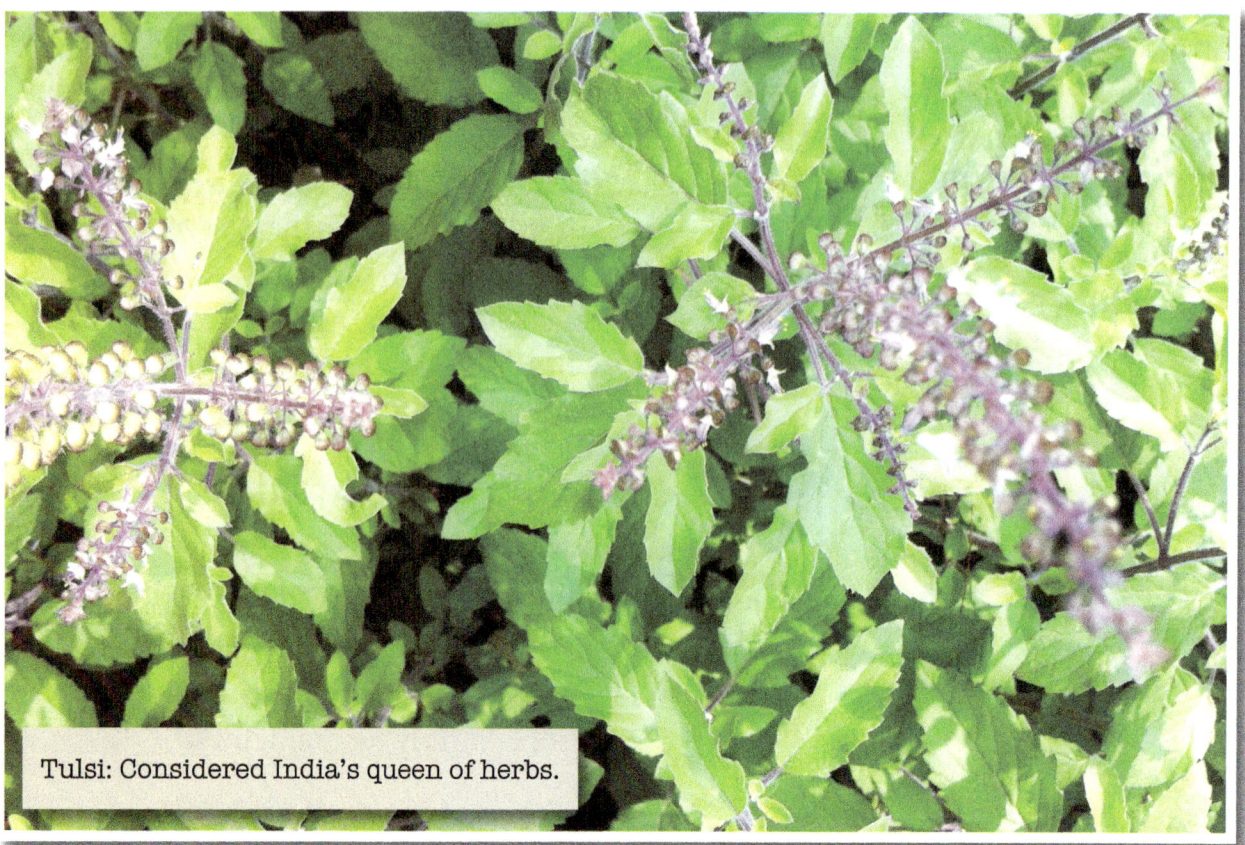

Tulsi: Considered India's queen of herbs.

Your Kitchen Apothecary

Establishing your own kitchen apothecary is a fun, easy and powerful thing to do.

I have found there is so much I can do at home to empower myself and my family when it comes to our health and healing. For peace of mind, we always consult our family doctor when our children are unwell. None of these remedies are meant to be a substitute for conventional medicine, however, they can work beautifully hand in hand.

Always use home remedies in consultation with your doctor.

For colds and flu, I love how effective a cup of chicken soup with a squeeze of lemon can be. Team that with a good dollop of raw garlic butter and we have nuked colds in record time.

For children older than 12 months, a dry cough is often relieved with a teaspoon of raw honey.

Tummy upsets are settled with warming lemon verbena teas, sweetened with raw honey.

Dehydration that comes about due to gastro is helped along with home made electrolyte drinks, jellies and icypoles made with coconut water, honey and herbal tea. You can even whizz up some watermelon or mango to sweeten the deal.

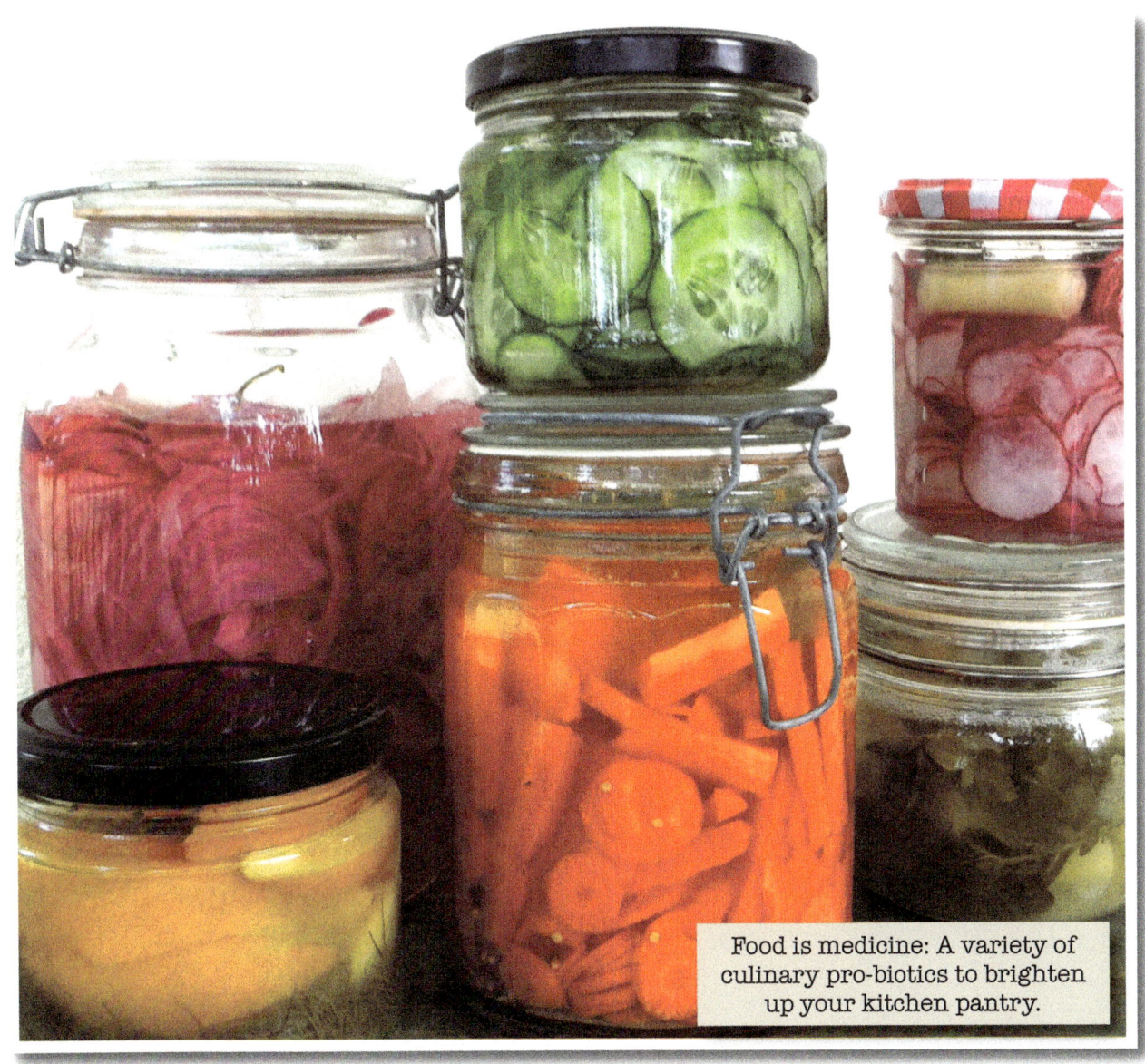

Food is medicine: A variety of culinary pro-biotics to brighten up your kitchen pantry.

Getting started

Stock your Pantry

I always have on hand:

Himalayan, Celtic or Macrobiotic salt
Apple cider vinegar with the mother
Raw honey
Cold pressed virgin coconut oil
Cold pressed virgin olive oil
Lemons/limes
Garlic
Ginger
Turmeric
Onions
Great Lakes Gelatine
Ghee
Variety of fermented foods
Bicarb of Soda
Epsom salts

Freezer

Chicken stock
Lamb stock
Garlic and herb butter
Frozen spray-free berries

My refrigerator is always full of:

Home made 24 hr yoghurt
Home made 24 hr cultured cream
Home made coconut yoghurt
Grass fed butter
Duck fat
Variety of fermented foods and drinks
Culture starter. I use Body Ecology or Caldwell's - both which can be found online.

My favourite fermented foods are:

Sauerkraut
Kimchi
Spanish onions
Dilly carrots
Dilly beans
Fennel
Beetroot and apple relish
Beetroot kvass
Water and milk kefir
Kombucha

When it comes to herbs, spices and healing, my favourites are:

Lemon verbena
Lemon basil
Sweet basil
Holy basil
Thyme
Oregano
Marjoram
Sage
Tarragon
Lemongrass
Parsley
Micro Greens
Coriander
Basil
Tumeric
Lemon balm
Hibicus
Gooseberry

Vegetable Patch/Pots

No matter what size garden you have a vegetable patch or pots are both a pleasure and a health plus.

I have had consistent success with:

Silverbeet
Kale
Zucchini
Beans
Peas
Strawberries
Peas
Broccoli
Radish

All culinary herbs are wonderful healers and easy to grow. Try them on a window sill or if you are really limited for space join a community garden or check out the power of sprouts. Broccoli sprouts in particular are known to have incredible anti-inflammatory properties.

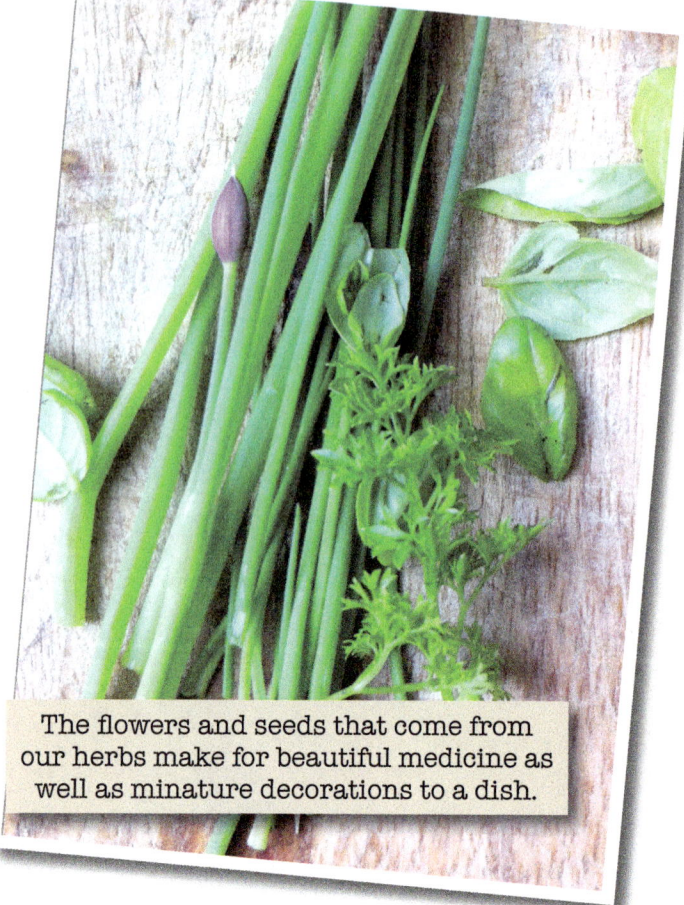

The flowers and seeds that come from our herbs make for beautiful medicine as well as minature decorations to a dish.

> Whenever possible we have a herb and vegetable garden growing. The kids love the fairy-tale quality of finding beans in their very own beanstalk.

The Basics

Garlic: Antibiotic, anti-inflammatory and anti-fungal.

Cultured cream

Boost your health one beautiful meal at a time. Do not underestimate the power of fat.

If you don't believe me just ask the French who seem to be quite partial to a bit of cream. My take is to culture the cream or make crème fraiche.

Turns out, studies have shown that if you add a bit of fat to your fruit it will help you to absorb the nutrients in the fruit. It will also slow down the sweet hit.

Ingredients

- Best quality 300ml cream
- ½ packet culture starter or 1 tbs of whey (I used Body Ecology)
- Filtered water

Making it

1. Get the best quality cream you can find and warm it gently on the stove. You should be able to keep your pinky finger in the cream for 10 seconds.
2. Add culture starter and a little bit of filtered water to a sterilised jar with an airtight lid.
3. Add the cream and give it a shake.
4. Wrap the jar in a tea towel and place it in an esky or cooler with a hot water bottle for 24 hours. Make sure you change the hot water bottle a few times over the 24 hours.

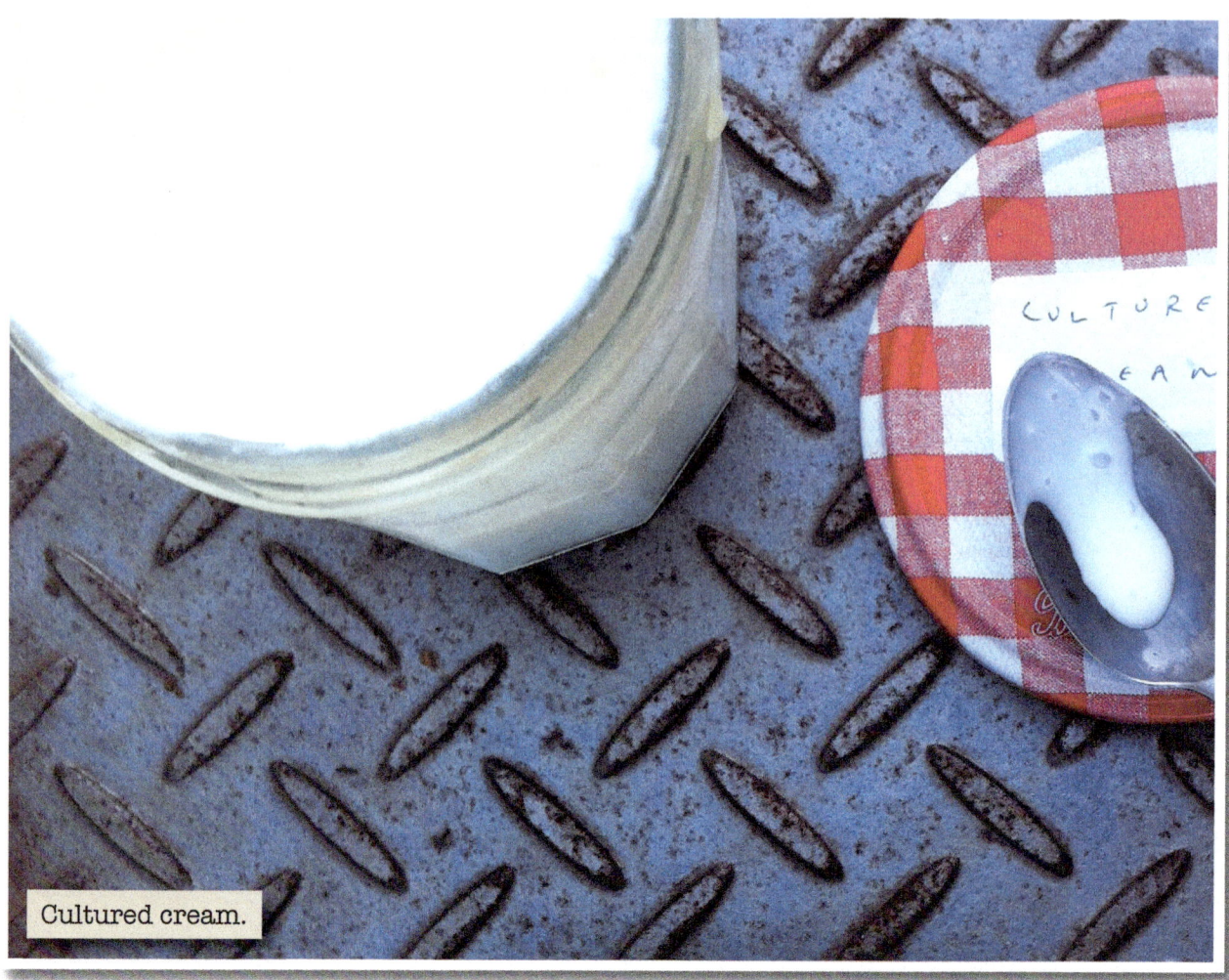

Cultured cream.

Yoghurt

Making our own yoghurt is surprisingly easy and fun.

The results are pretty yummy too.

If you eat a lot of it in your house it will be considerably cheaper for you to make as well.

The key to it is that you need to introduce a small amount of the yogurt you like to make more of it. You can then reserve a little of the yoghurt you have made to make your next batch.

> We do a 24-hour ferment, which is said to help remove the bulk of the lactose within the milk – something that is problematic for many with digestive problems.

Ingredients

- 1 litre of organic, full cream milk.
- 4 tbs of organic full cream Greek yoghurt.
- 1 tbs of cream (optional)

Making it

1. Heat milk until just about to boil but do not let it get to that point. You should have tiny little bubbles forming on the side but nothing hotter than that.
2. People use thermometres, but I didn't have one so I just went with the old school method. Many cultures have been making yoghurt by feel for centuries.
3. Have your sink ready with cold water and submerge your pot of milk in the water to allow it to cool quickly.
4. You should be able to put your pinky in it for about 10 seconds. It's important to get to these temps so that a culture can grow when you add it.
5. Add the yogurt culture and stir but do not over stir. You can even add a good dollop of double cream, which will give it an amazing rich, thick quality.
6. Pour contents into sterilised glass jars and put somewhere warm so culture can grow. I got a hot water bottle filled with warm water and put it in an esky with a blanket over the top.
7. You need about 24 hours to let the culture develop and your yogurt is nice and thick. Then refrigerate for a few hours. It will thicken as it gets colder.

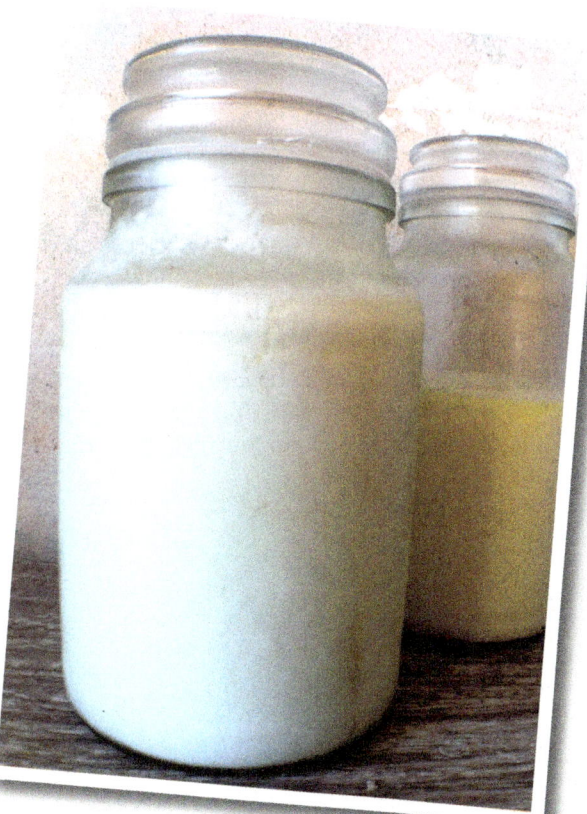

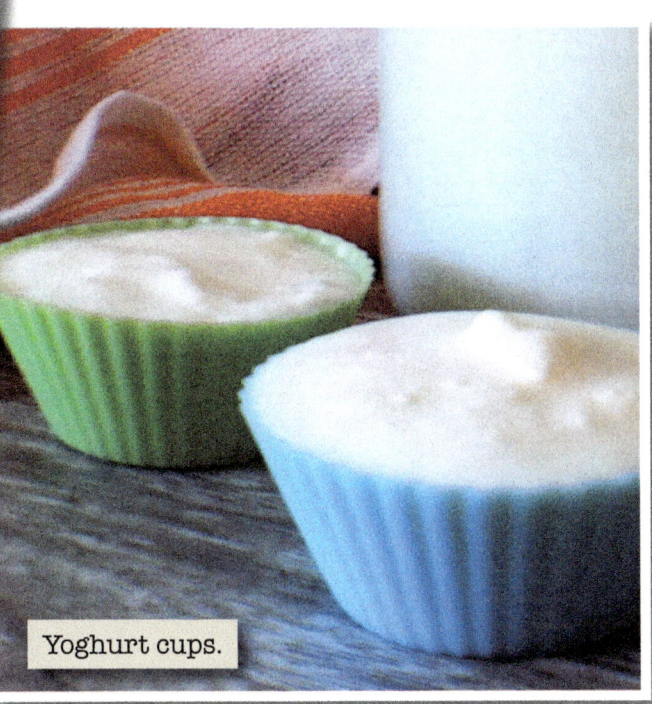

Yoghurt cups.

The mighty chicken stock

It was Grandma's cold remedy, a comfort food, an old-school staple and something no top restaurant would ever be without.

These days, many buy it in a cardboard box to boost the flavour of their meals but what if I told you that home made chicken stock was one of the most powerful healing foods I have come across to date?

Simple to do, super cheap - just put it all in a slow cooker for a few hours and forget about it.

The result: A nutrient dense food, packed with properties which are perfect to help soothe inflamed gut lining.

When you boil meat on the bone for a long period of time you will draw out the gelatine.

High in collagen, gelatine is said to help heal and seal a leaky gut - a condition according to neurologist and nutritionist Dr Natasha Campbell McBride, which can cause many allergies and neurological conditions.

Gelatine contains glycine which can promote sleep and calm nerves among other things. The collagen within gelatine is a natural beauty product to boot.

We make sure to have a cup a day. The whole family has it - even our dog Lexi has been put onto an onion and garlic free version.

> We discovered that stock was right for our dog after vet visits and carprofen failed to help her arthritic limp. We were delighted to see her running limp-free after a few weeks of stock and regular doses of apple cider vinegar in her water bowl.

Ingredients

- One whole chicken, or any good quality meat with bones if you want a lamb, fish or beef stock. (organic is always preferred but do what you can afford).
- 1 shallot or onion, 1 leek, 3 garlic cloves, 1 celery stick and 2 carrots
- 1 tbs apple cider vinegar
- 1 tsp sea salt

Making it

1. Put the salt and the vegetables listed above - or any combination of your favourite vegetables - into a stock-pot or slow cooker along with the chicken.
2. Cover with filtered water and put on a slow simmer with the lid on for at least three hours if using the stockpot. If using a slow-cooker put it on for at least eight hours.
3. The stock can be strained, or enjoyed as a soup.
4. Reserve the chicken for another meal.
5. By following the same method, the chicken bones can be reused and made into a mineral-packed bone broth, which is said to be rich in calcium. This is an advanced food for some. Simmer gently for about 8 - 24 hours for best results.

Extra tips

We put some apple cider vinegar in ours - my mum puts in a heap of spring onions - which is yum.

We freeze a good portion in ice trays and use them daily.

For an Asian inspired stock, try adding lemongrass, ginger, kaffir lime leaves, Vietnamese mint, garlic and Chinese five-spice. This makes a wonderful gift for a new mother or anyone who is under the weather.

For economy and extra flavour, use the carcass of a roasted chicken with some meat still on it. Boil it along with any remaining fats, veggies and lemon you might have stuffed the chicken with.

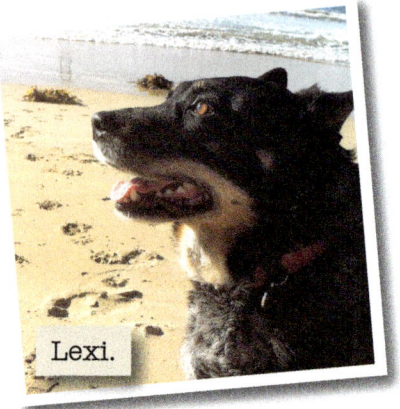

Lexi.

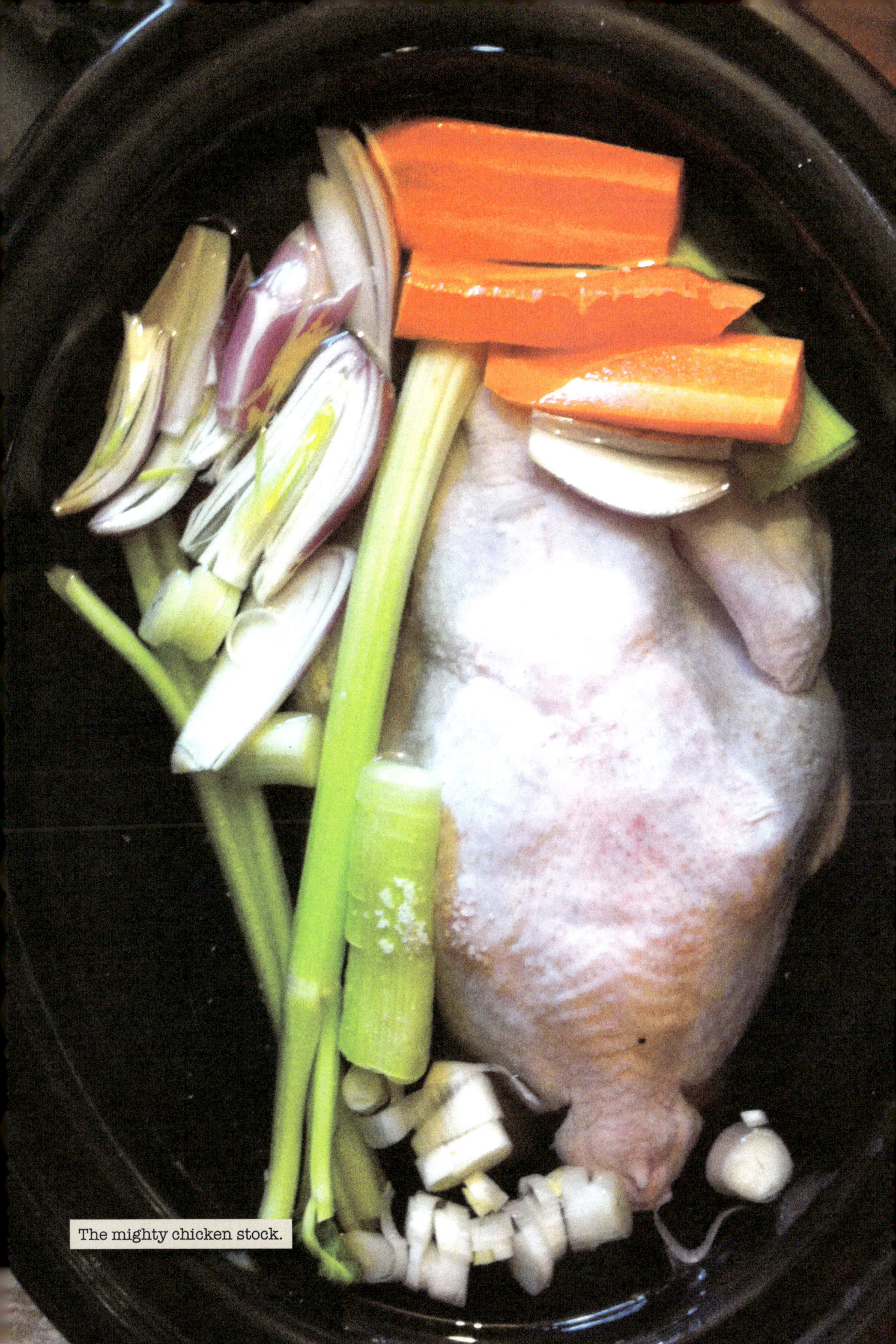
The mighty chicken stock.

Condiments

It's easy to change up the flavour of your meals by adding a new condiment.

Try these combinations by whizzing the ingredients together in a food processor or a stick mixer.

Egg-free aioli

Ingredients

- 2 tbs olive oil
- ½ cup cultured cream/home made yoghurt or coconut milk
- Two roast garlic cloves
- 1 teaspoon home made mustard
- ½ tsp raw honey
- Lemon or lime zest.

Salad dressing

Ingredients

- 2 tbs olive oil
- 1 teaspoon apple cider vinegar
- A squeeze of lemon.

Avocado salsa

Ingredients

- Half an avocado
- Handful of fresh parsley leaves, stalks removed
- A good slug of olive oil
- Pinch of good quality mineral salt
- A squeeze of lemon
- Half a diced tomato
- Add roasted or raw garlic cloves if you have them.

For an Asian variation blend together spring onions, Vietnamese mint, Coriander, Olive oil, 1 teaspoon of finely grated fresh ginger, 1 clove of pressed garlic

Omega 3 rich sauce

Ingredients

- 2 tbs olive oil
- ½ tsp raw honey
- 1 tsp apple cider vinegar
- A squeeze of lemon
- 3 sardines fillets preserved in olive oil.

Nut free pesto

Ingredients

- 2 tbs olive oil
- A squeeze of lemon
- 1 tbs chopped soft herbs (basil is traditionally used, but parsley, or coriander also work beautifully)
- 1tbs Parmesan cheese (omit if dairy intolerant).

Yoghurt mint dip

Ingredients

- A squeeze of lemon
- 1 tbs chopped mint
- 1 cup of yoghurt
- ¼ clove of pressed raw garlic
- Finish with a slug of olive oil.

Home made mustard

Ingredients

- ⅓ cup mustard seeds
- ⅓ cup apple cider vinegar
- 1 tablespoon raw honey
- 1 teaspoon ground turmeric
- ½ teaspoon Himalayan sea salt
- 2-4 tablespoons of warm water

1. Place ingredients in a glass jar with a lid and let stand. Cover, and let stand for 2-3 days.

2. Empty contents of the jar into a plastic jug. Whiz until as smooth as possible. Add water if the mustard is too thick.

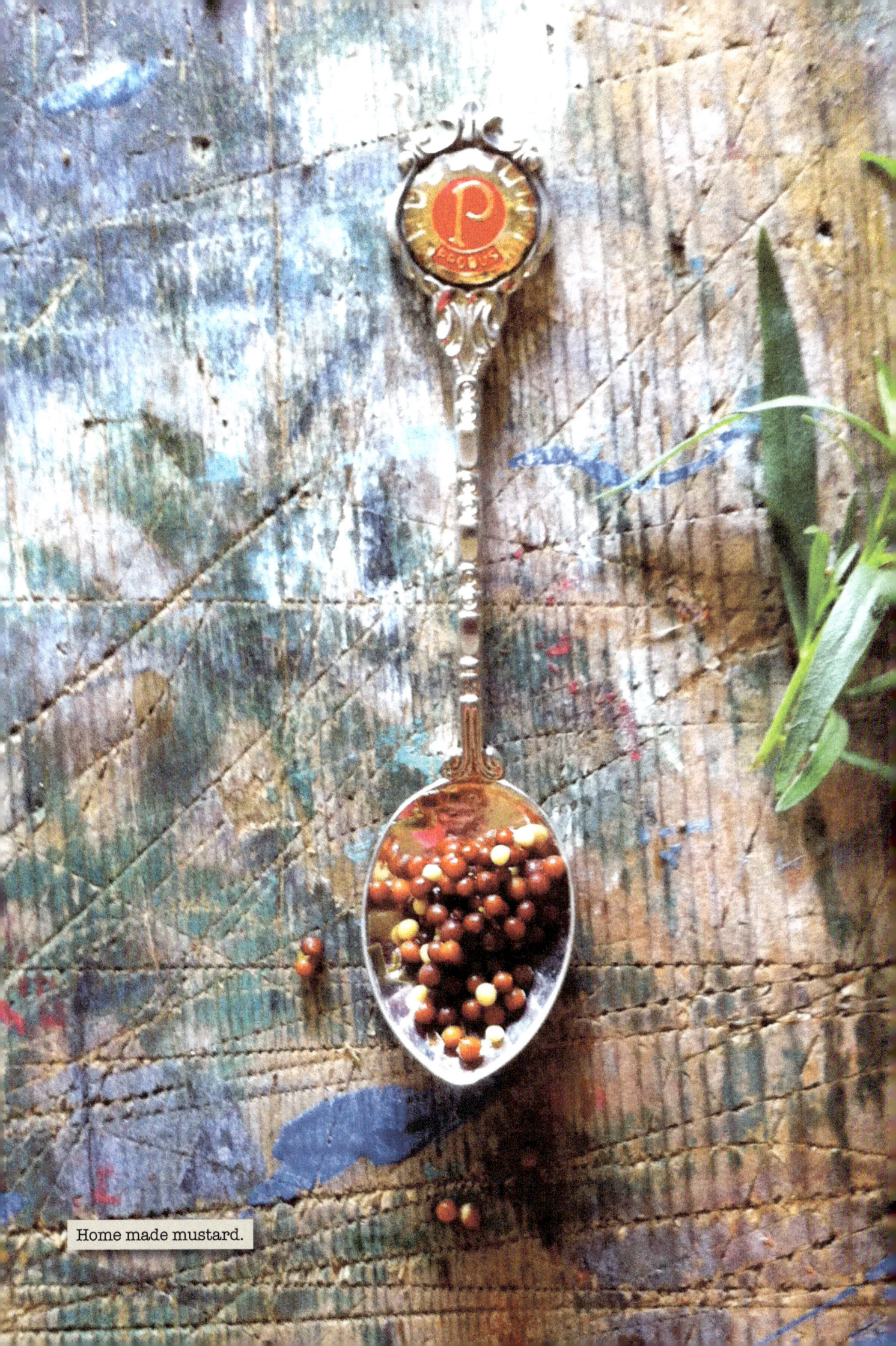

Home made mustard.

Salts

Salts: Empires have been built on the stuff.

It's a vital ingredient in cooking but also for preserving food. In our little household a pinch of good quality salt goes into all of our cooking.

> This morning, my girls and I made a few different salts together. It's fun to see them pound the crystals into fine grains and make something I know they are going to love sprinkling on their food.

I find the more involved they are in the cooking process, the more likely they are to try new things.

Sumac, lemon & thyme salt

Ingredients
- 1 cup Himalayan salt crystals
- 2 tsp sumac
- 1 sprig lemon thyme
- 1 tsp finely chopped dried lemon rind

Making it
1. Pound all ingredients together in a mortar and pestle until salt crystals are fine and sumac evenly distributed.

Extra tips

Sumac salts are one of many blends I make when I get on a roll. I love giving these as presents and I'm always on the look out in op shops for pretty little crystal salt mills which look so lovely on your kitchen bench.

I don't normally measure when making them up but more go by the feel, taste and look of things.

I always keep a box of Himalayan salt crystals on hand – they need to be big so you can use your mortar and pestle to grind them with your herbs.

Dried will work best – but experiment with what you have around you. I just invent more and more with them with whatever I had on hand. I recently even put some dried rose petals and orange rind in one of my salts.

On this day particular day, I had a dried up old lemon so I cut the skin off and chopped it up into tiny little pieces. Anything goes.

We love: Rosemary salt, Lemon and chilli salt and French Sel de Provence (Traditionally this would be a mix of oregano, thyme, basil, sage, rosemary and lavender flowers).

All herb salts take only a few minutes to grind together.

Do about a tsp of the herb or spice of your choice to half a cup of salt crystals.

I have some purple sage growing so I might try that next...

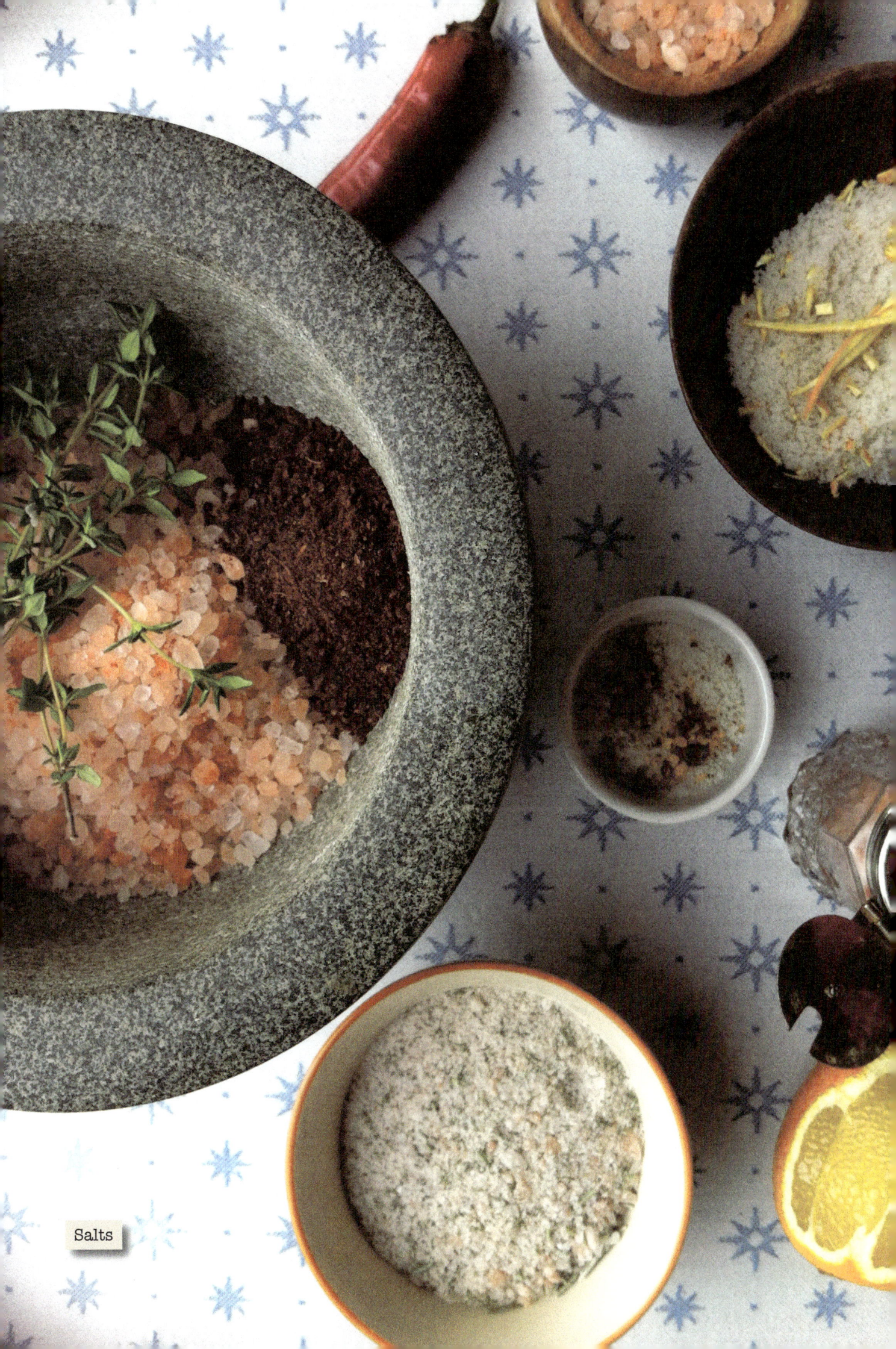

Salts

Vanilla orange rind extract

I thought it would be nice to have some home made vanilla extract – one without sugar.

I had a bottle of vodka and some organic oranges. I cut off the skin being careful not to include the pith (white part). I then added a couple of vanilla beans.

Ingredients
- 2 cups vodka
- 4 vanilla beans
- 1 tbs of orange rind cut into fine strips.

Making it
1. Rind of half an organic orange sliced finely
2. Pack into a glass jar and allow it to sit in a dark cupboard for three months.

Extra tip

You will know when it is ready because the vodka will take on a lovely dark caramel colour. The extract will smell distinctly of orange and vanilla.

For variation, do a mint extract using about a cup of fresh mint from the garden. This will go well with chocolaty desserts. Also, don't forget to do a plain vanilla extract. Perfect to have on hand. Perfect to give as a gift.

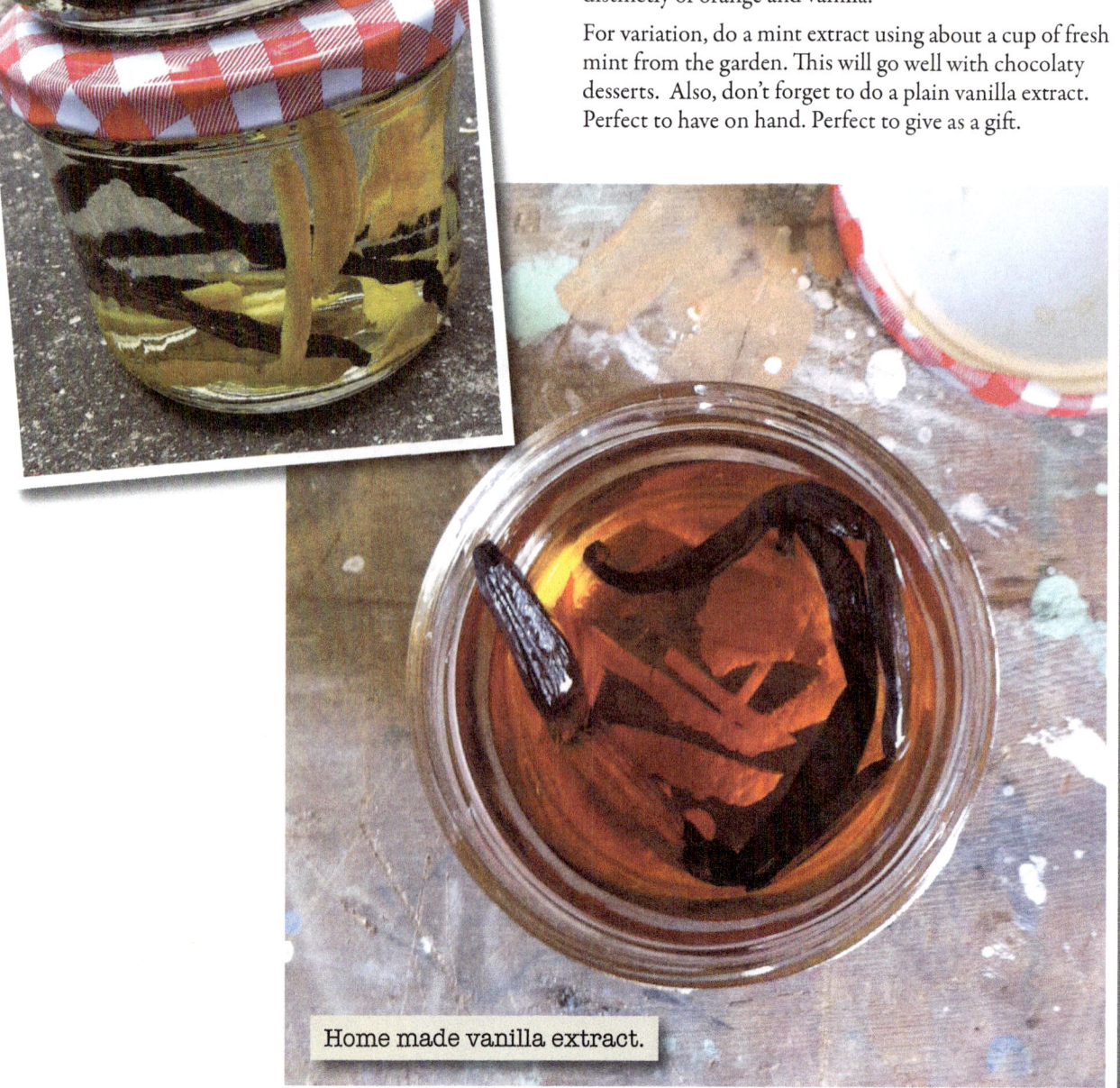

Home made vanilla extract.

Culinary Probiotics

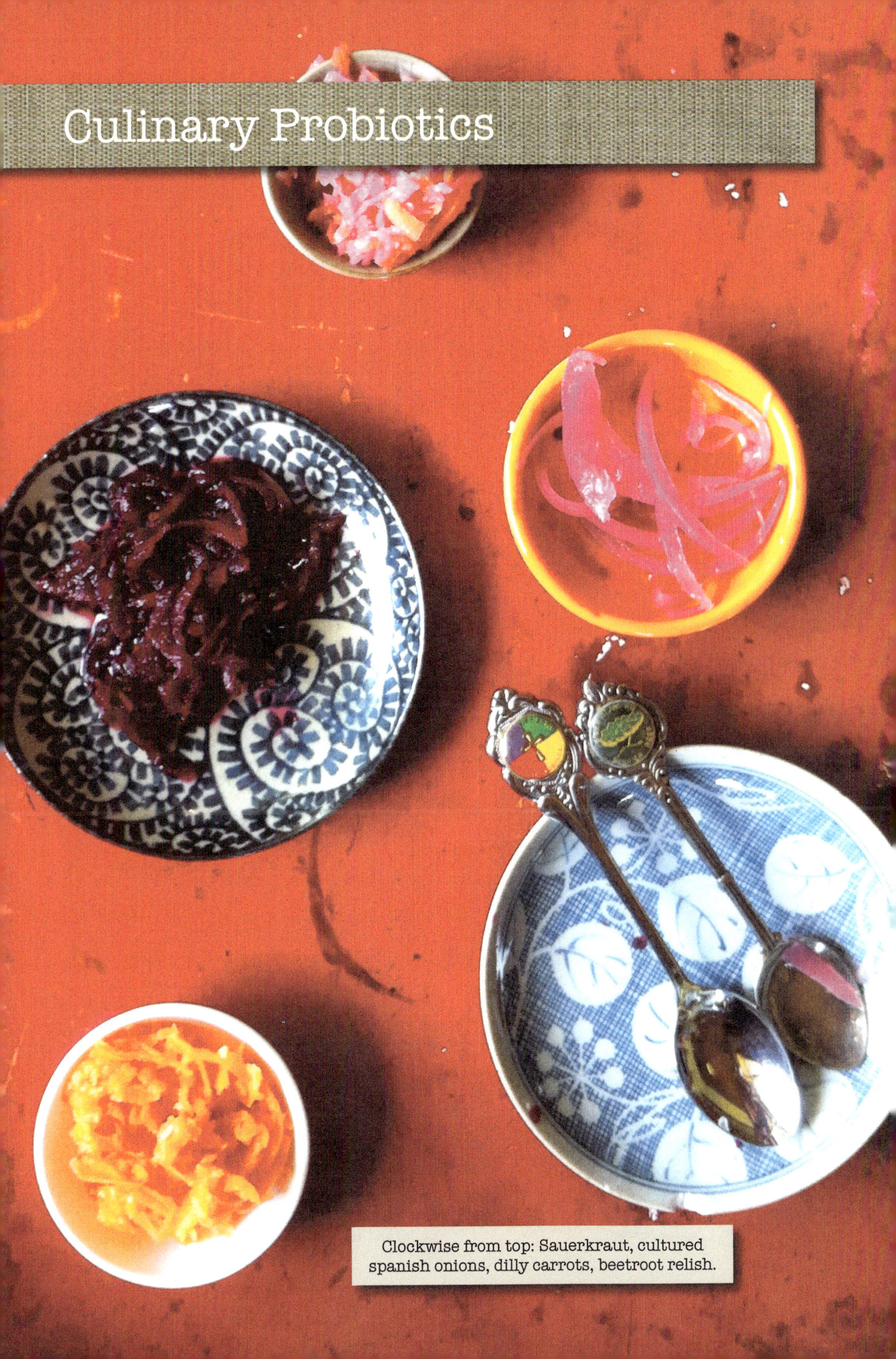

Clockwise from top: Sauerkraut, cultured spanish onions, dilly carrots, beetroot relish.

Fermented foods

Fermented food has been a revelation for us and a vital part of Stevie Rose's healing.

Thanks to her, we all now make sure we have a spoonful of something fermented with every meal wherever possible.

The process of lacto-fermentation is a way of helping to correct the balance of good and bad bacteria living in the gut.

When gut problems arise, often a large part of the cause is due to an overgrowth of bad bacteria.

Whether it be strep, clostridia or yeast - the list goes on - the most effective way to get things under control is to slowly and systematically crowd out these bugs until things are back in balance.

> When we first started on ferments, the histamines in them affected Stevie a lot. She experienced a lot of what is known as 'die off' which is physical and emotional discomfort when the bad bugs start to be brought back into line.

I suppose the easiest comparison I can think of is if you've ever given up coffee. You can get a headache and feel cranky, your body can ache...it's a similar phenomenon.

Because of this, we quite literally started on a drop of sauerkraut water a day at a time.

Slowly and painstakingly, we gently built up to a point where now histamine sensitivity has been eliminated and delicious servings of fermented foods are unlimited

I am truly thankful to our Australian ferment queen and GAPS consultant, Kitsa Yanniotis, of Kitsa's Kitchen who makes this beautiful food for the public to buy.

Find her at: http://www.kitsaskitchen.com.au

We used her products initially while I was learning to make our own with great results.

This way, unfamiliar with the flavours of fermented food, I was able to get a sense of how they should taste and she then helped enormously by giving me tips and tricks on how to ferment correctly.

Some fermentation basics

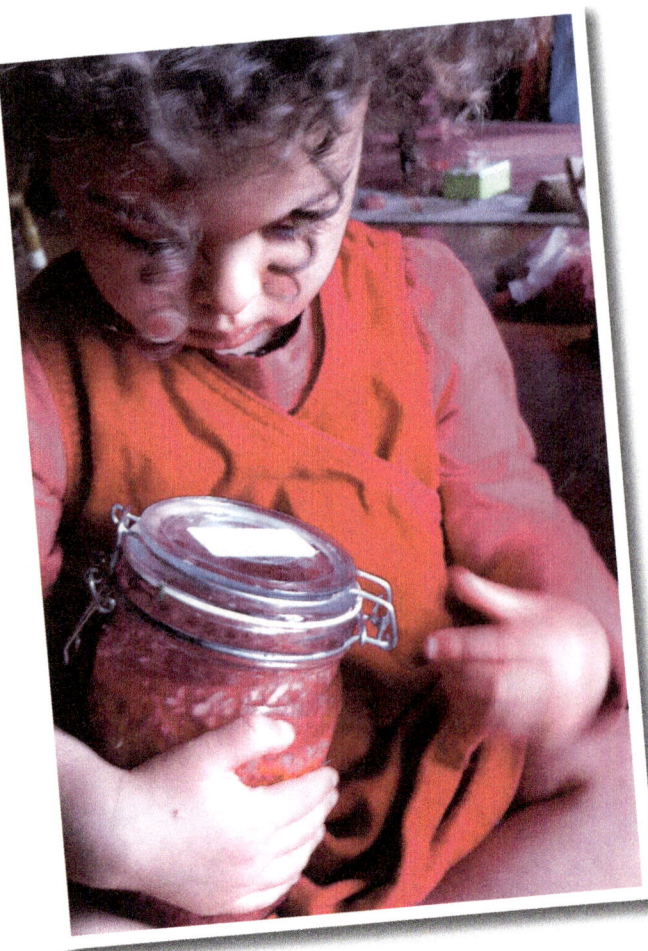

When fermenting at home I have had good success with Fido jars, or clip down lids with a rubber seal. This allows for the slow release of gas during the fermentation process.

The right salt is also important. I use Himalayan, Celtic or Macrobiotic salt found in our local health food shop. I haven't found success with ordinary table salt. The iodine is apparently problematic.

Filtered water is also important. Chlorine is said to interrupt the fermentation process. I use a bench top sized Britta jug, which works well for us.

When fermenting vegetables I like to work on a 2 per cent salinity ratio of salt to water. That generally amounts to 1 teaspoon of salt to every cup of water used.

Be sure to sterilise your jars and have a clean kitchen before beginning. I often clean jars by using hot soapy water and rinsing and drying thoroughly with paper towel. Others like to finish with a few minutes in a warm oven.

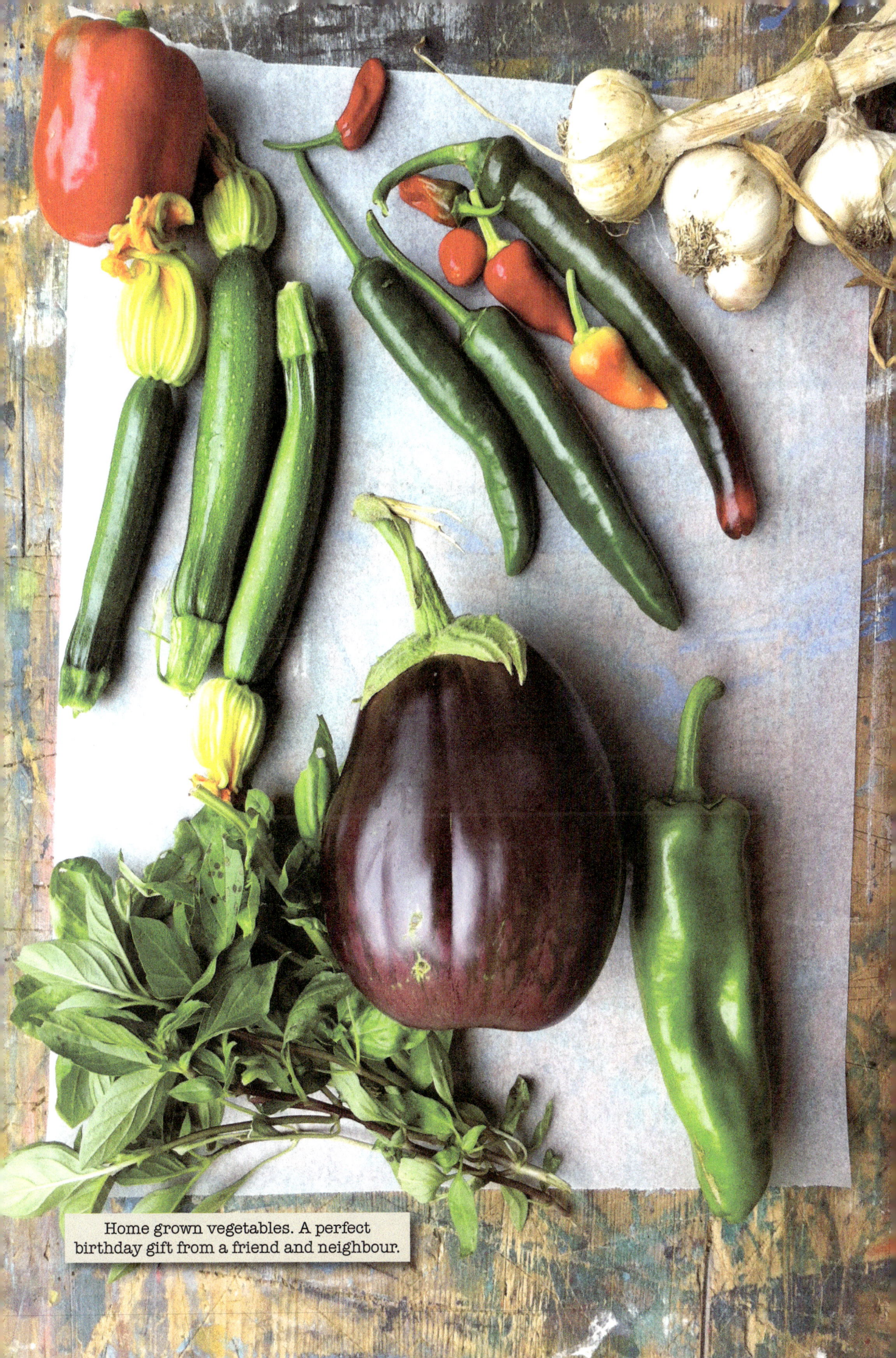

Home grown vegetables. A perfect birthday gift from a friend and neighbour.

Sauerkraut - master technique

This is the mother of all ferments.

Super-rich in Vitamin C, an immune system booster, sauerkraut works like a digestive enzyme helping send down an army of helpers into your tummy to help you digest your meal.

Ingredients

- 2 organic cabbages, one red, one green
- 2 large organic carrots
- 2 tbs good quality sea salt, plus more for brine (you can add culture starter but it is not essential).
- ½ tsp caraway, dill, or fennel seeds (optional).
- 1 large glass jar (about 3 litres) with a clip down lid.
- Filtered water (culture will not grow using chlorinated water).

Making it

1. Take outer leaves off and reserve the cleanest one for later. Cut the head into quarters and remove the core. Finely chop using a food processor if you have one.

2. Put cabbage in a large bowl, and toss with 2 tsp sea salt. Using a wooden spoon, pound the cabbage for a few minutes to help release the natural juices.

3. Put into your sterilised glass jar. Layer cabbage with carrot and then purple cabbage - this will turn it a very pretty pink colour. Pack the vegetables in the jar nice and tight but only until the shoulder.

4. Make additional brine water to top up jar until it covers the veggies. To do this, dissolve the remaining salt into two cups of room-temperature filtered water. Pour this into the jars until the cabbage is covered. Fold up your outside cabbage leaf and put it on top of your veggies to weigh them down. You don't want them to come above the water.

5. Close your lid, wrap it up so it doesn't get into any direct sunlight and give it 14 days. After this time, take the top leaf off and any darkened veggies.

6. Kraut gets better as it matures in the fridge. Will keep for many months.

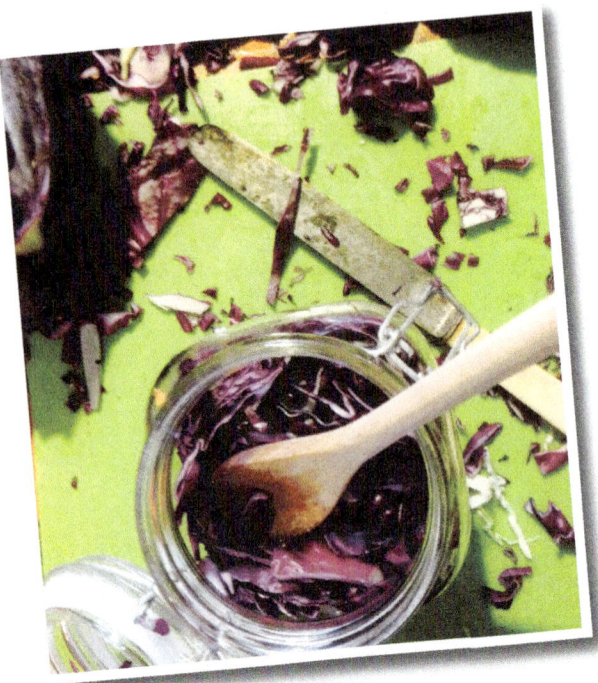

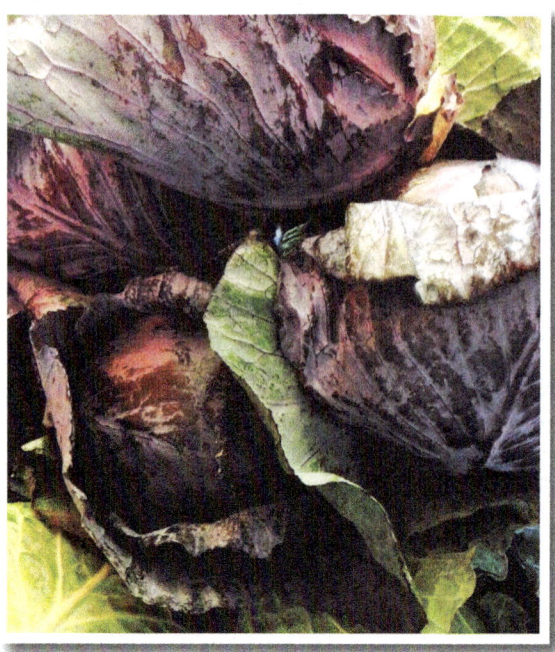

I find some ferments need a weight to keep the vegetables submerged under the brine while others don't. This prevents spoilage during the process. The cabbage leaf can be a great option but I have also used glass weights, a small ceramic dish, or even celery sticks cut length ways to fit the jars. The celery sticks must be submerged under the brine for them to be effective.

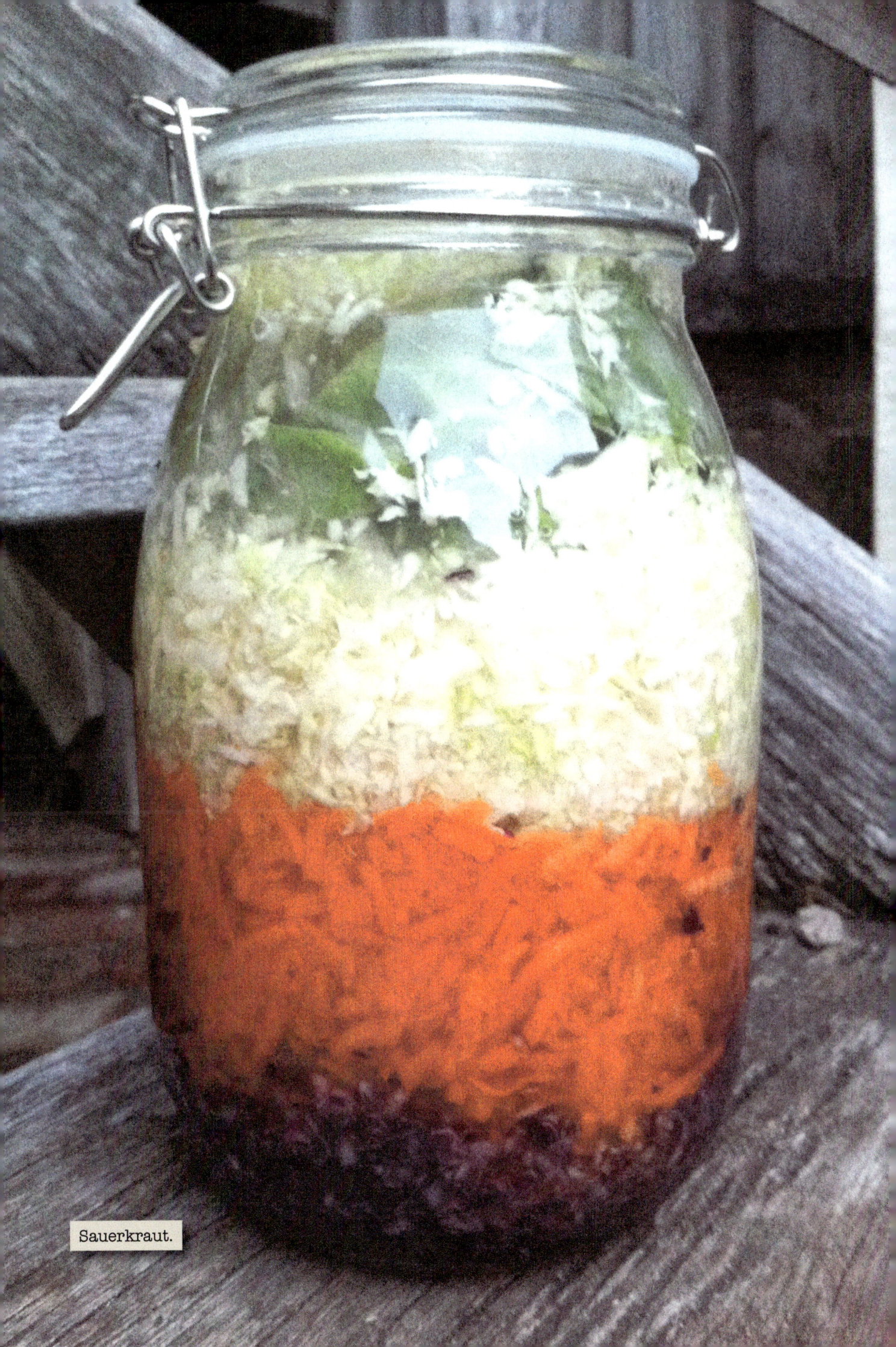

Sauerkraut.

Fermented garlic

Fermented garlic is a great way of getting a super charged hit of anti-inflammatory, anti-fungal goodness.

Most children dislike the burney quality of raw garlic however if you ferment cloves for a while, they lose their sharpness.

I always find squeezing garlic cloves through a press takes the edge off and fermenting them with beetroot provides a lovely purple disguise as well as a sweet beetrooty flavour.

Ingredients

- 3 large bulbs of garlic, peeled
- 3 stalks thyme or oregano
- 1 tsp fresh lemon rind (optional)
- 1 tsp Himalayan, Celtic or Macrobiotic salt

Making it

1. In a 500 ml capacity glass, flip top jar, fill the cloves into the jar up to the shoulder and cover with filtered water.
2. Add about a teaspoon of salt
3. Add thyme or oregano and lemon rind if desired
4. Leave to ferment for about two months. Garlic should be firm but have lost much of its hot quality when you taste it.

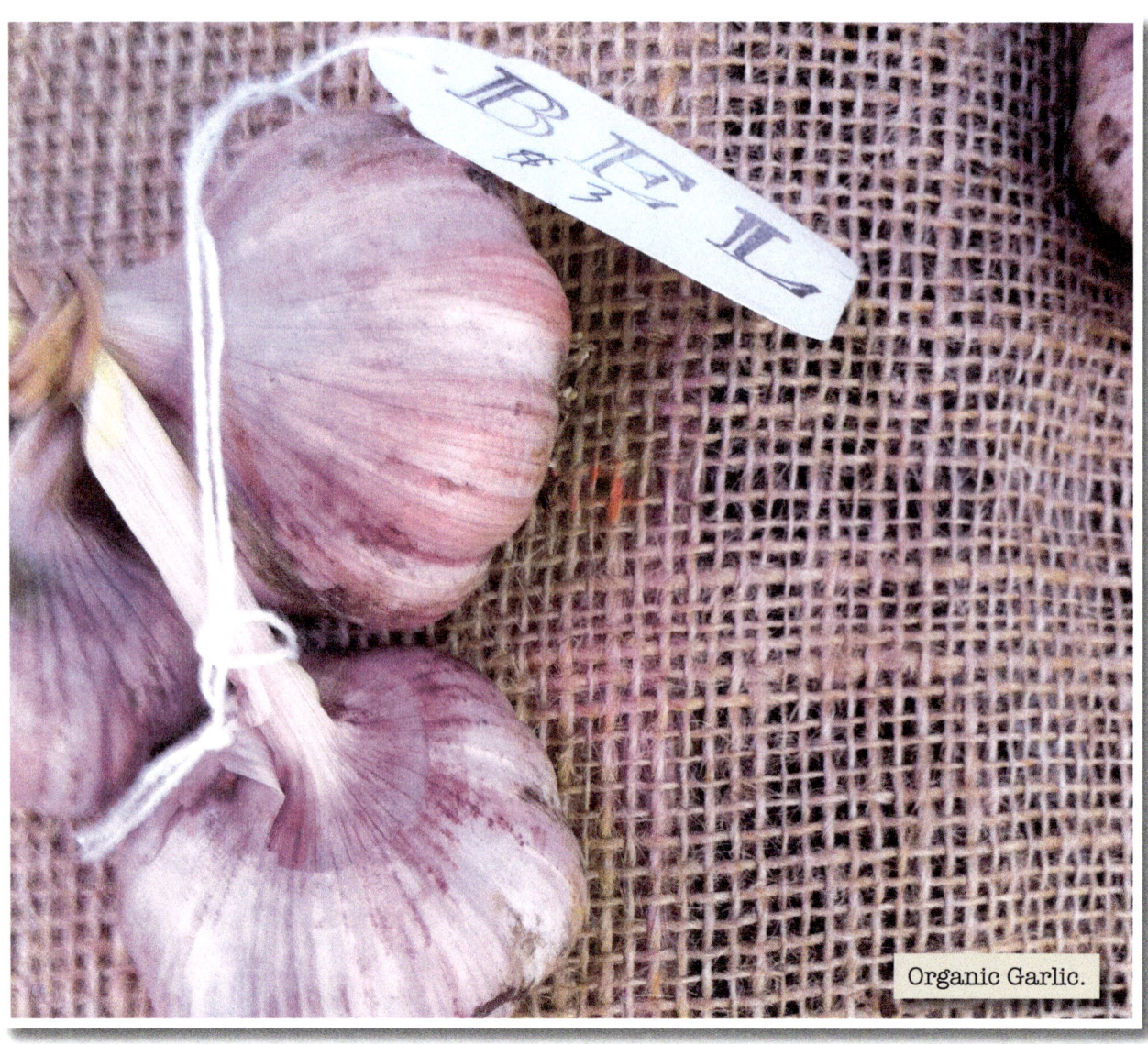

Organic Garlic.

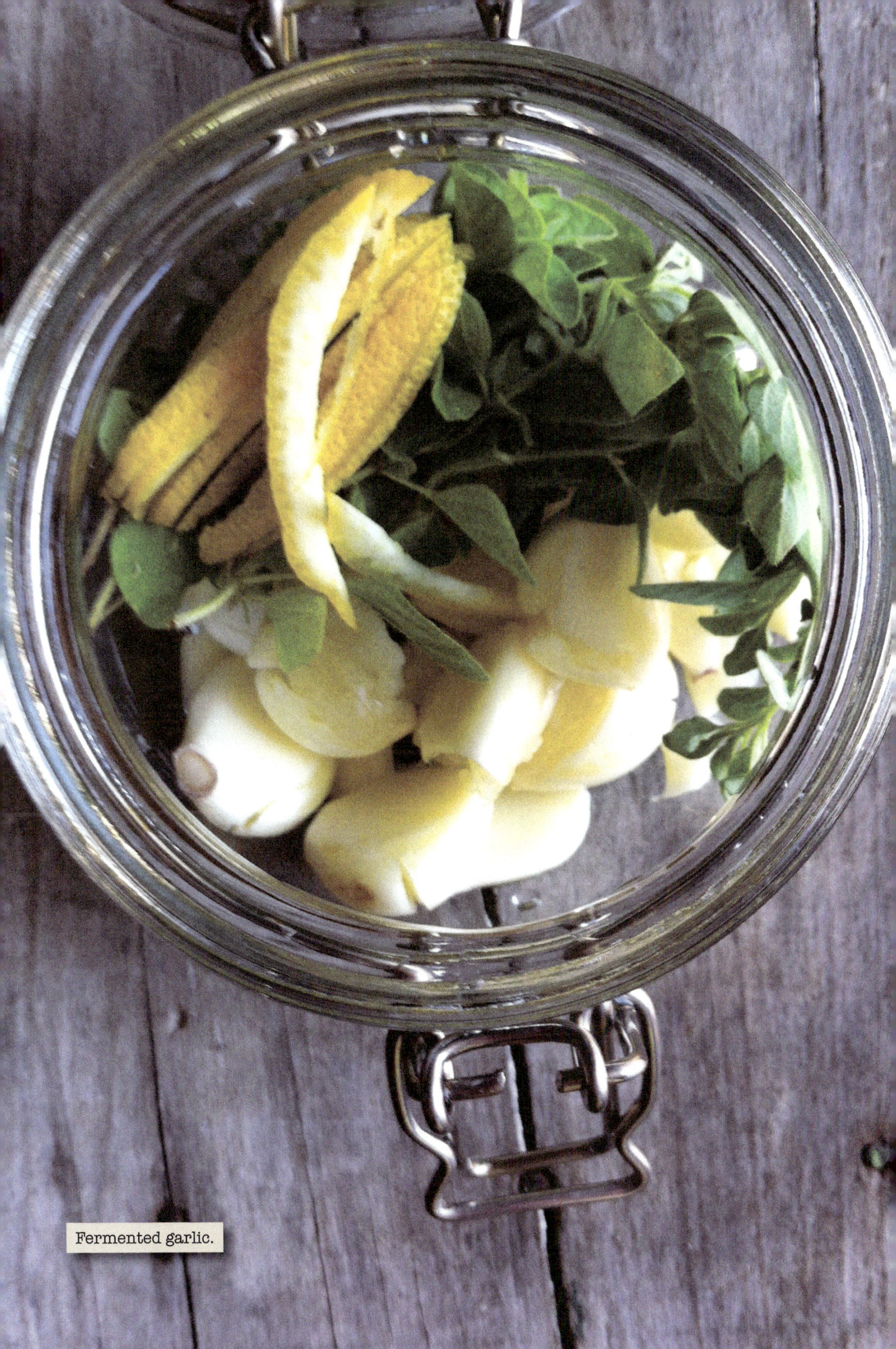
Fermented garlic.

Radish with kaffir lime leaves

This is a light, summery ferment that makes for a great condiment if you are having any kind of fish.

It's peppery taste is lovely mixed through a salad. It is also, I realise, a favourite food of the rhinoceros.

Ingredients

- Eight radishes thinly sliced
- 1 tsp Himalayan, Celtic or Macrobiotic salt
- 1 Kaffir lime leaf (you can sub for thyme if you wish)

Making it

1. Take a bunch of radishes and slice finely with a mandolin or even peel with a potato peeler to make sure they are super fine.
2. Place in a jar that is about 500 ml.
3. To this, add one kaffir lime leaf. This is a beautiful, generous tree to have growing in your garden or in a pot if you have the space.
4. Fill to the shoulder of your glass jar and add one teaspoon of good quality sea salt.
5. Pound the radishes with a wooden spoon for about a minute to release the juices and then fill to cover the vegetables with filtered water.
6. Cover tightly and leave in a warm place in your kitchen, away from direct sunlight for three days.
7. Transfer to the fridge and give it about three days to develop.

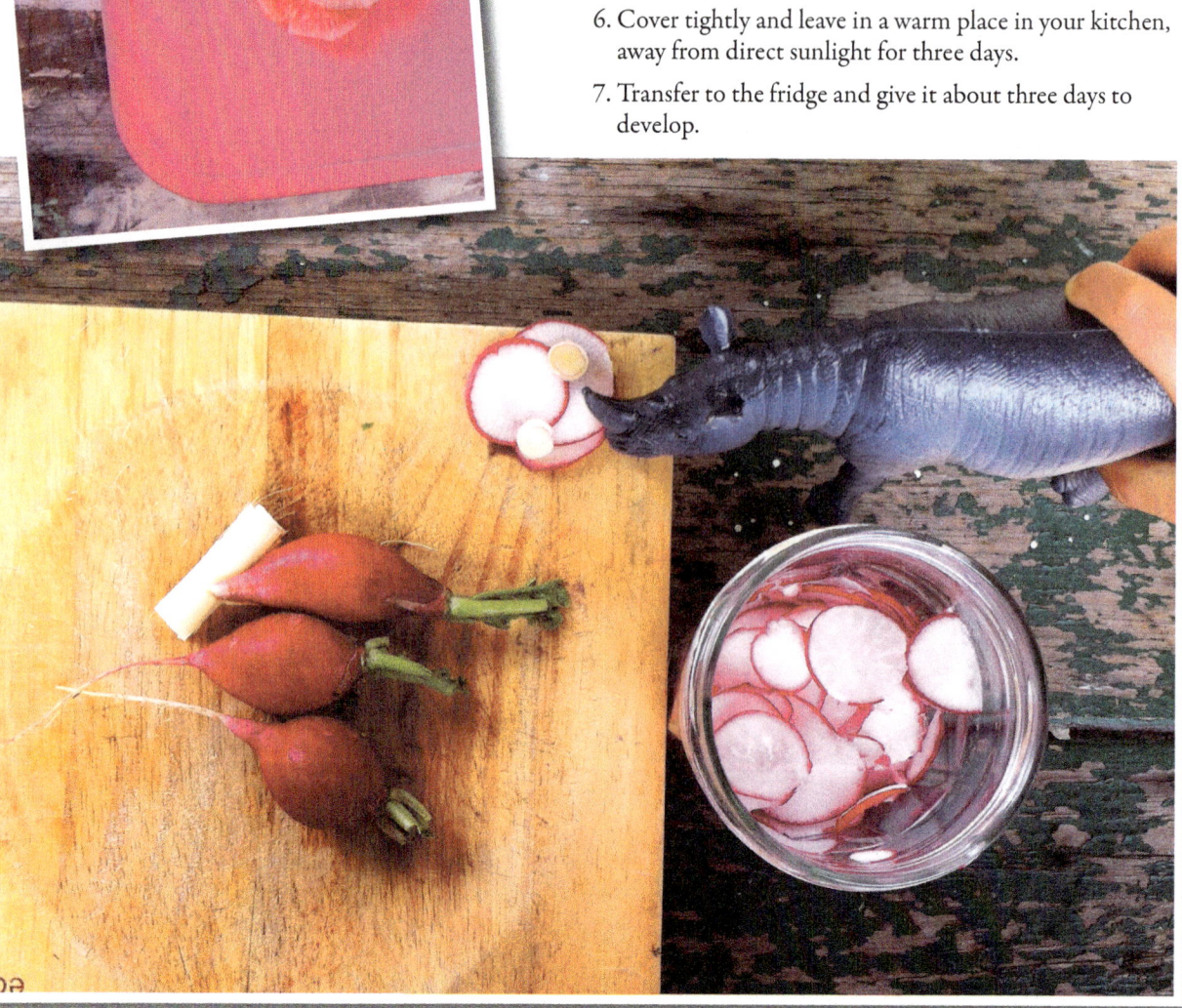

Dilly sliced cucumbers

Getting these right was surprisingly difficult. It's about getting your salt ratio right.

Also, I finally realised the tannins in grape leaves are paramount to getting that crunchy, fresh, sour/salty flavour that everyone loves about pickled cucumber.

This tip comes thanks to the godfather of fermentation Sandor Katz. Check out his book *Wild Fermentation* for a full run down on his beautiful philosophy.

Ingredients

- 2 Lebanese cucumbers
- 1 grape leaf
- 1 tsp Himalayan, Celtic or Macrobiotic salt
- 1 tsp dill or parsley seeds

Making it

1. Take organic Lebanese cucumbers and slice finely with a mandolin or a sharp knife. Place in a jar that is about 500 ml.
2. Add dill or parsley seeds.
3. Fill to the shoulder of your glass jar and add one teaspoon of good quality sea salt. Gently press the cucumber slices with a wooden spoon for about a minute to release the juices and then fill to cover with filtered water.
4. Cover tightly and leave in a warm place in your kitchen, away from direct sunlight for three days.

Transfer to the fridge and give it about three days to develop.

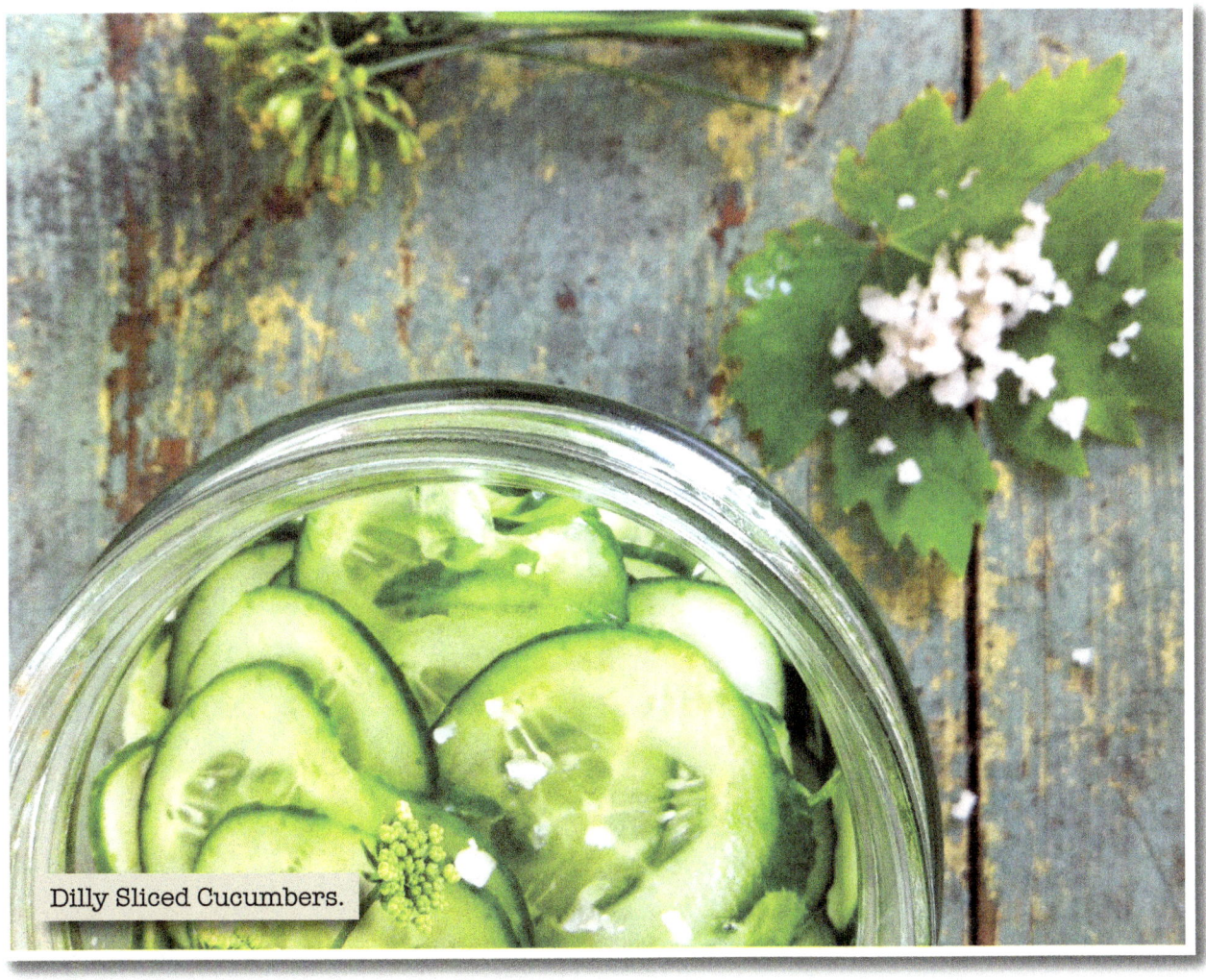

Dilly Sliced Cucumbers.

Middle Eastern beetroot & turnip mezze

Mezze is the shared small plates of food so popular in Middle Eastern, Greek and Spanish cultures.

Call it tapas or mezze, but no matter what culture you are referencing you can have many of your small plates ready to go well in advance, making putting on a lunch or dinner a snap.

I'm thinking, slow cooked lamb shoulder with cinnamon and orange rind on a wooden board; a bowl of warmed olives; a salad of green beans, preserved lemons, orange slices and lettuce from the garden; a yoghurt and mint dip; some sunflower seed crackers with paprika sprinkled on top and these ...

Ingredients

- 3 beets
- 2 turnips
- 2 cloves garlic
- 1 teaspoon of dill or fennel seed
- 2 tsps Himalayan, Celtic or Macrobiotic salt

Making it

1. Julienne beets and turnips in a food processor or using a mandolin.
2. Add the garlic cloves and herbs and mix together.
3. Place mix in a jar and periodically add sea salt or culture starter and pound with a wooden spoon to encourage the juices to release.
4. Fill your jar (about 1 lt capacity) with filtered water. Leave about 2cm of space at the top for the vegetables to bubble and expand as they culture.
5. Let your jar sit in your kitchen out of direct sunlight for about seven days.
6. Keep in the fridge.

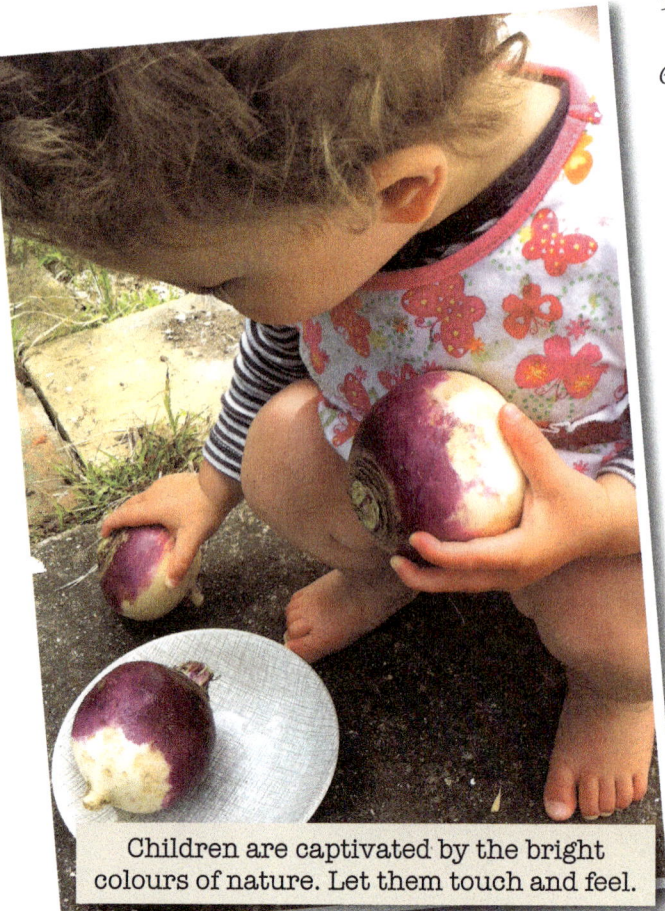

Children are captivated by the bright colours of nature. Let them touch and feel.

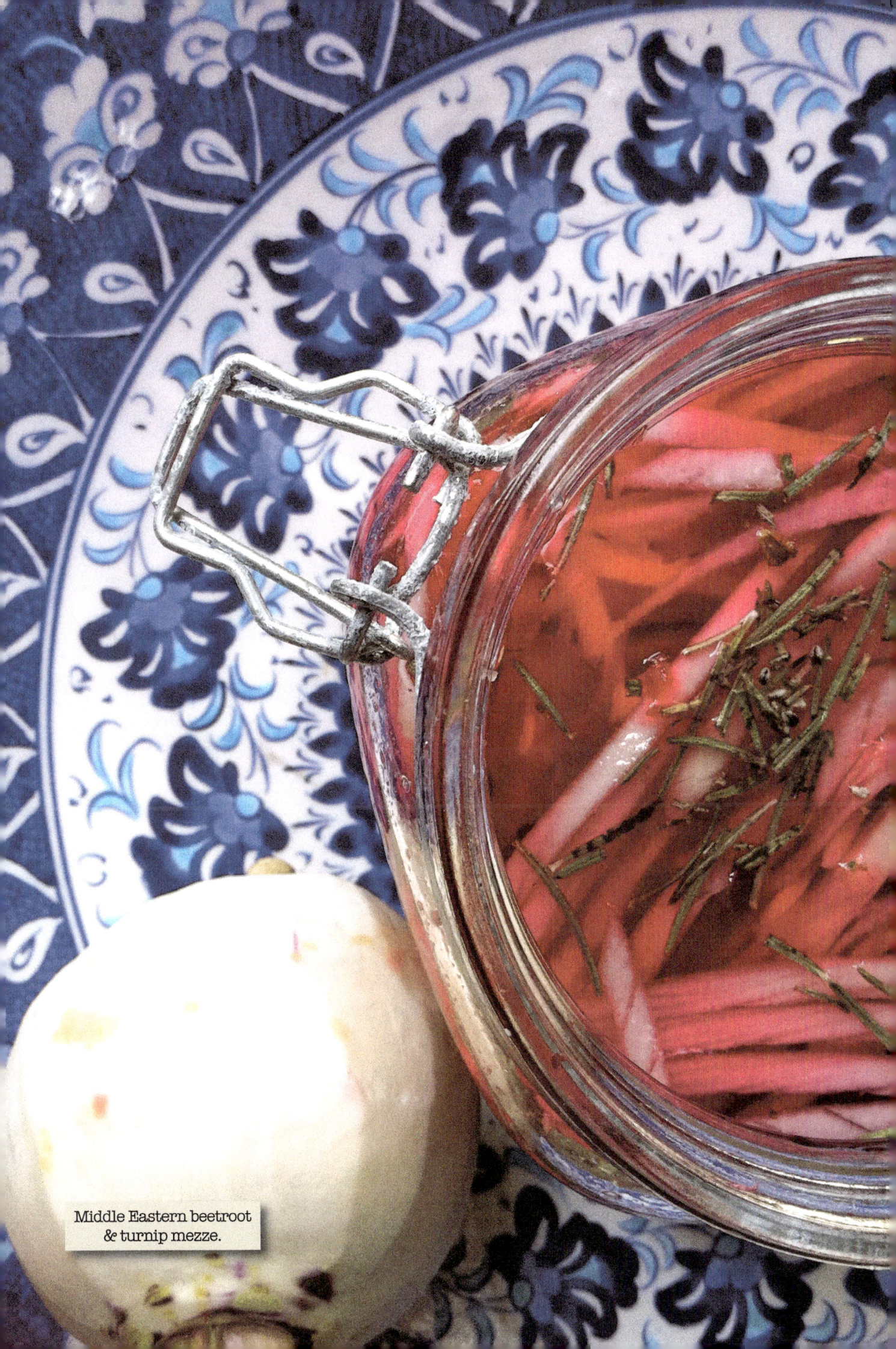

Middle Eastern beetroot & turnip mezze.

Carrots sticks with mustard seeds & garden herbs

Carrot sticks are often a great way to introduce children to the world of fermented food.

Sweet, sour and crunchy, these are great with a mint or avocado dip made with fermented garlic, coconut/cow/goat milk yoghurt and fresh herbs.

Ingredients

- Three organic carrots, peel and julienne
- Tsp of mustard seeds
- 1 tsp Himalayan, Celtic or Macrobiotic salt
- Two bay leaves (optional)
- Three sprigs of thyme some celery leaf, oregano and dill seeds (optional)

Making it

1. Place in a jar that is about 500 ml.
2. Add a teaspoon of mustard seeds, two bay leaves, three sprigs of thyme, some celery leaf, oregano and dill seeds.
3. Fill to the shoulder of your glass jar and add one teaspoon of good quality sea salt.
4. Pound the carrots with a wooden spoon for about a minute to release the juices and then fill to cover the vegetables with filtered water.
5. Cover tightly and leave in a warm place in your kitchen (your kitchen bench is ideal), away from direct sunlight (cover with a tea towel if you need to) for about five days.
6. Transfer to the fridge and give it about five days to develop.

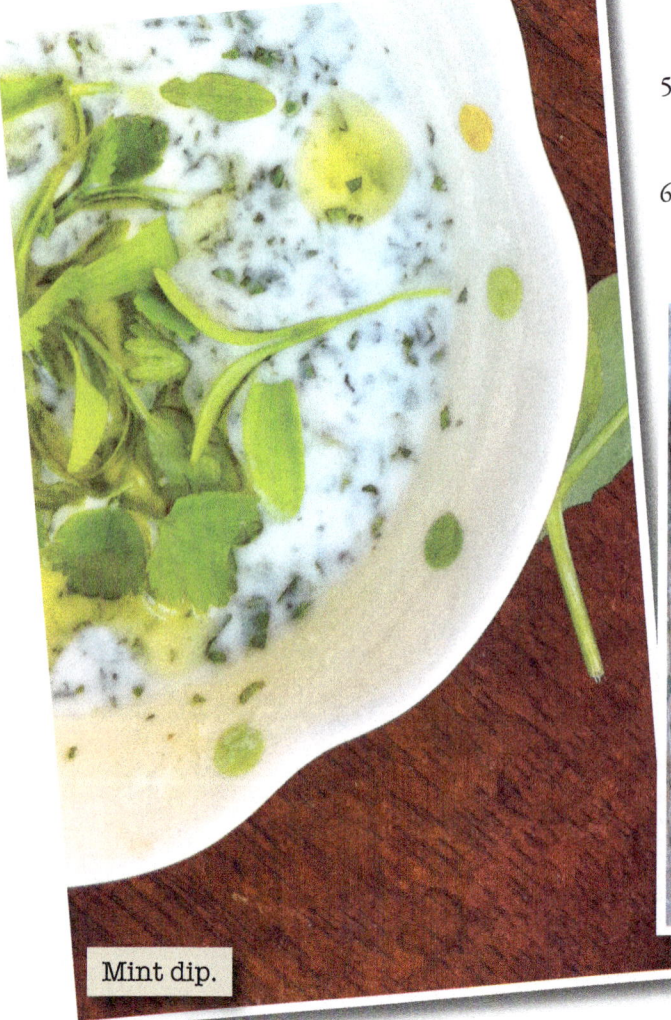

Mint dip.

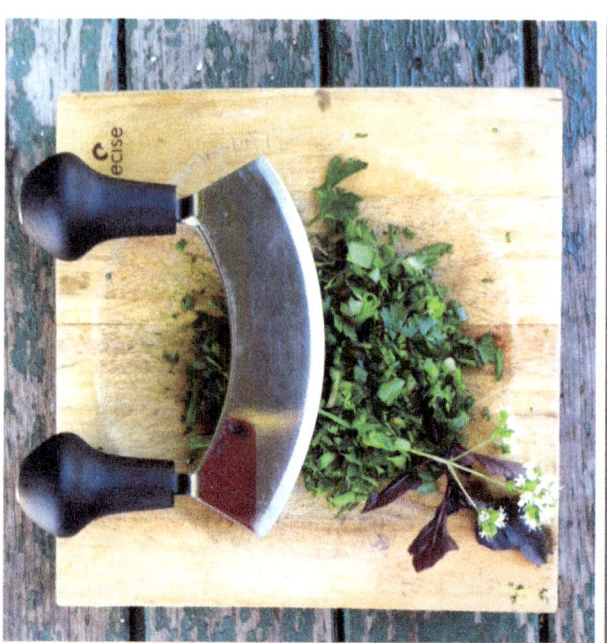

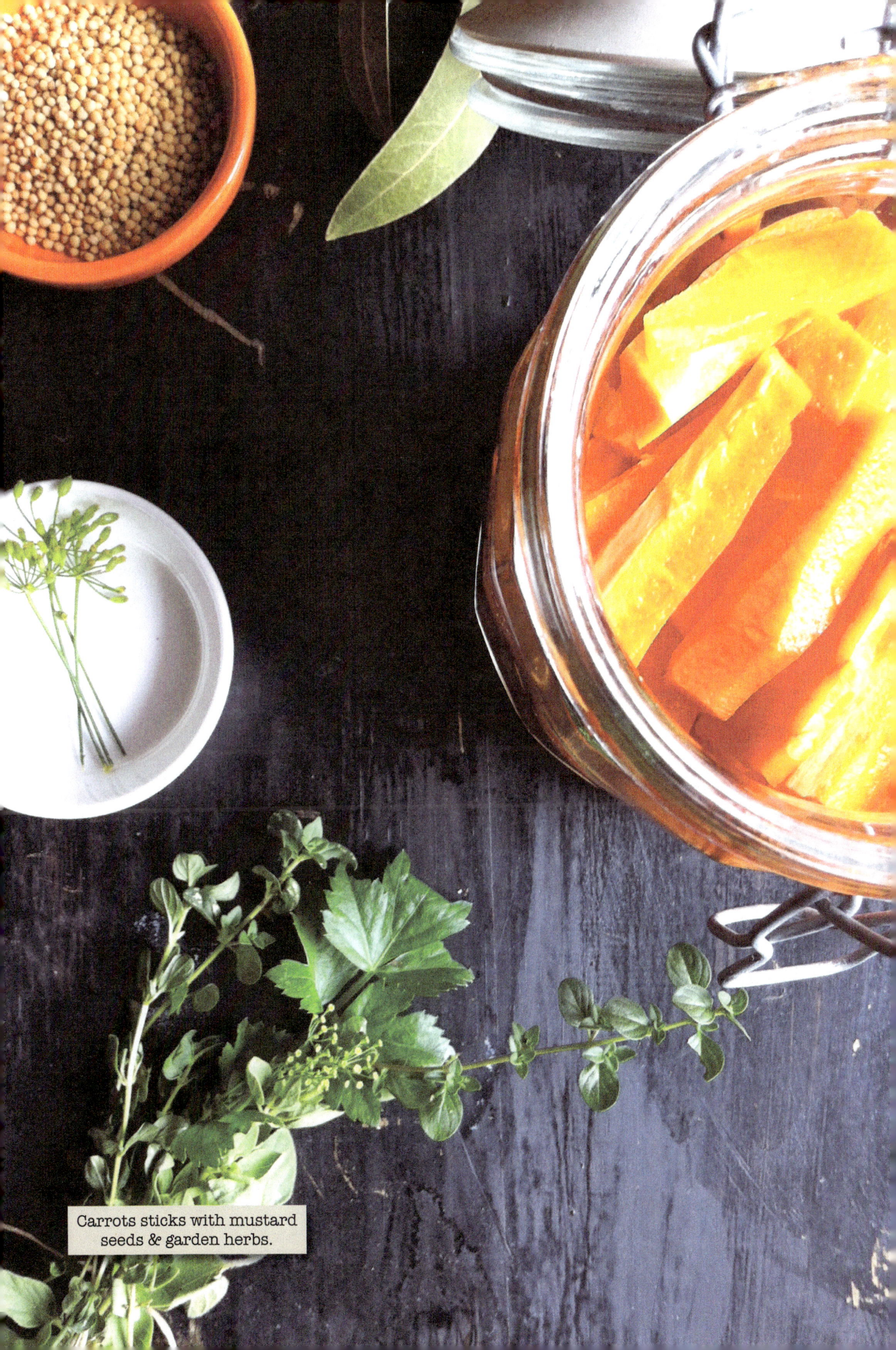

Carrots sticks with mustard seeds & garden herbs.

Spanish onion with thyme & garlic

Sweet and pungent, this ferment is great on top of home made baked beans, makes for a great side next to lamb and can be slipped into salads without getting your kids offside.

High in sulphur, they are great to help with detoxification, they are a good source of the anti-oxidant flavonoid quercetin, which has been found to have anti-carcinogenic, anti-inflammatory and anti-diabetic functions.

Ingredients

- 1 tsp of macrobiotic or Celtic Sea salt.
- 2 large Spanish onions
- 6 thyme sprigs
- 2 cloves garlic
- 1 tsp salt

Making it

1. Thinly slice the onion. Put the onion, thyme and garlic in a sterilised glass airtight jar - I used one that was about 500mls.
2. Add the culture and/or the salt and fill your jar with filtered water. Leave about 2cm of space at the top for the onion to bubble and expand as it cultures.
3. Let your jar sit in your kitchen out of direct sunlight for three days depending on the warmth of your kitchen.
4. Place in fridge to keep. It will get better and better with time and will keep for months.

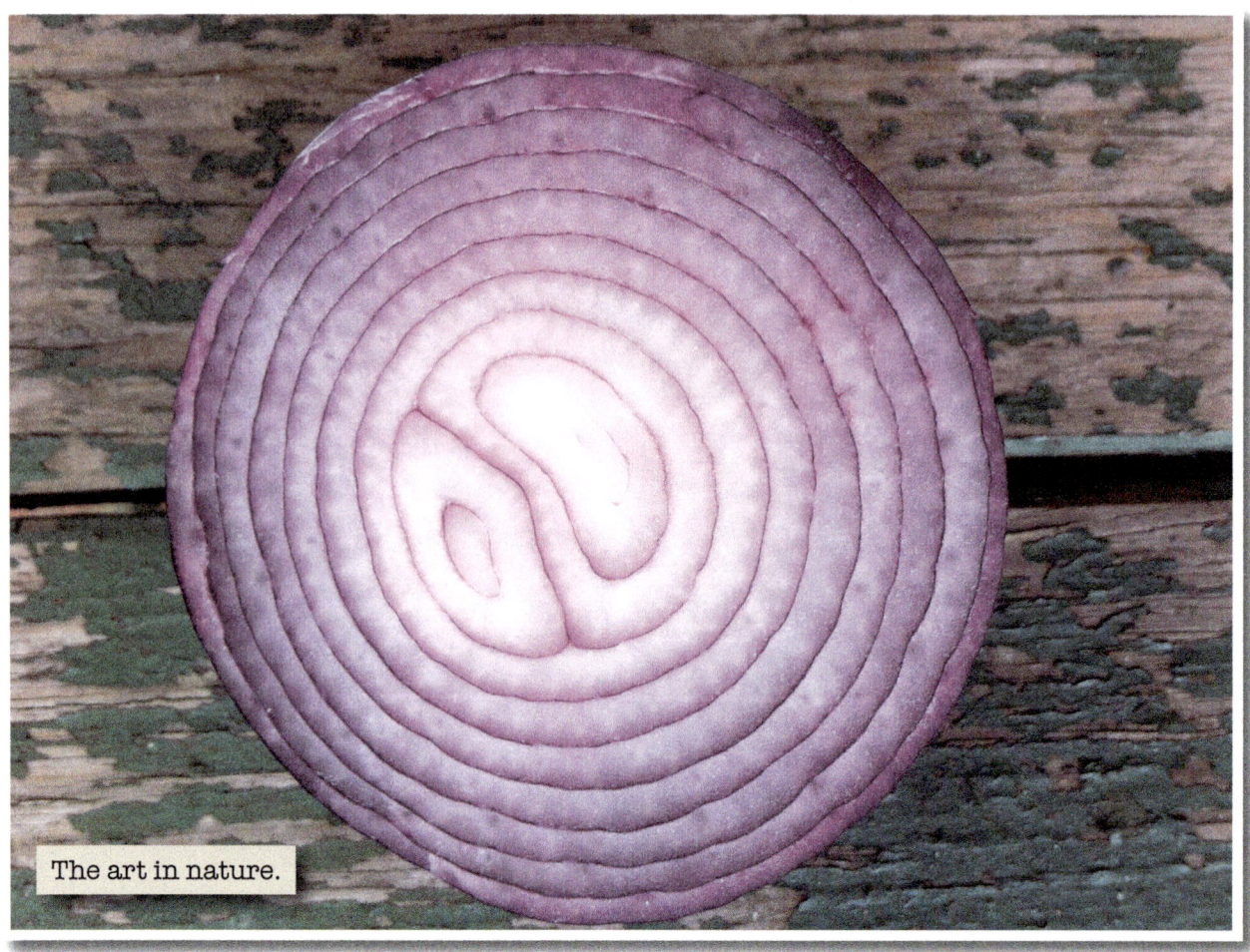

The art in nature.

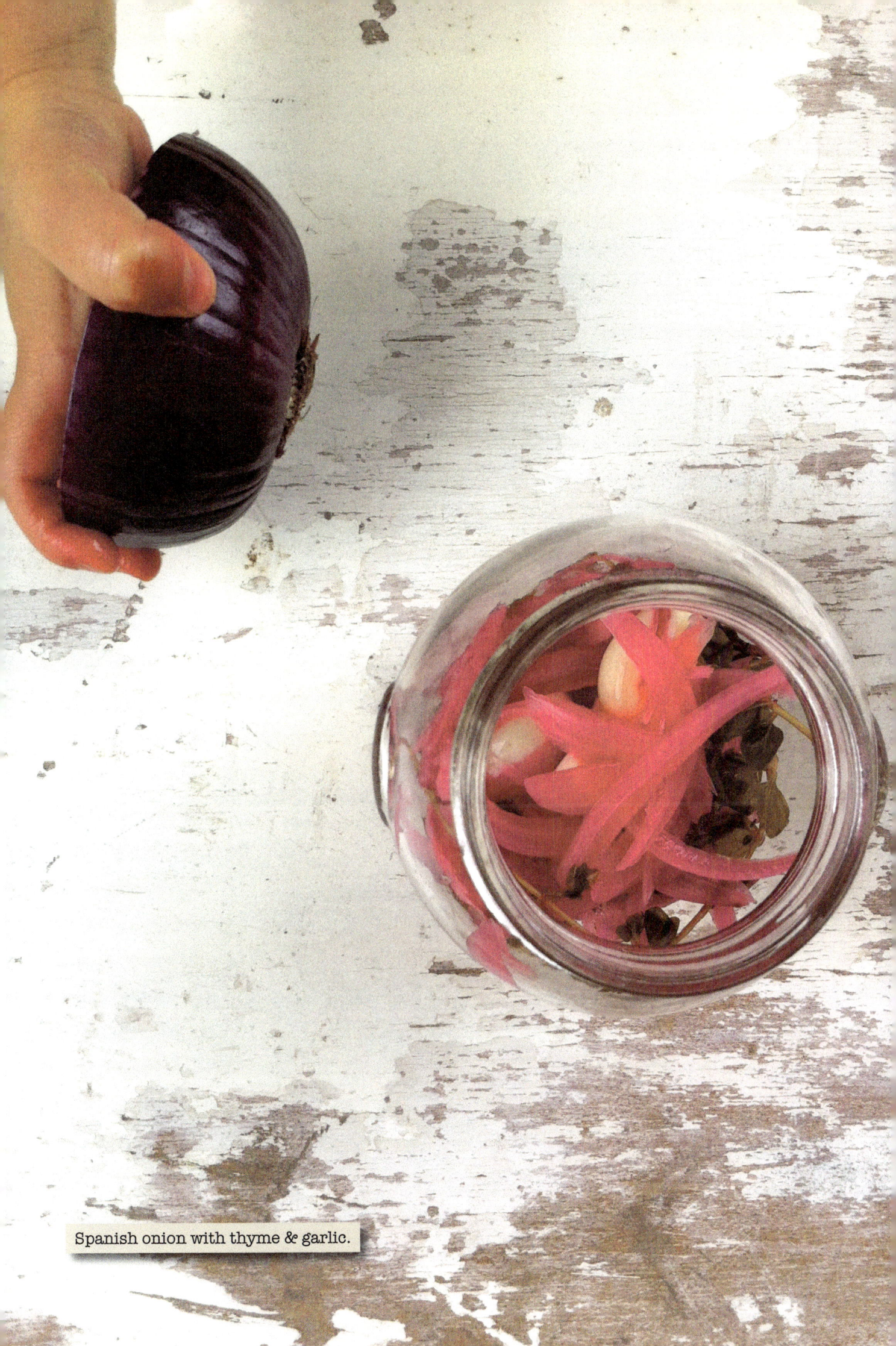

Spanish onion with thyme & garlic.

Fermented beetroot with turmeric, orange rind & cinnamon

Another great intro ferment for the littlies.

Beets are so sweet, they are also known in Chinese Medicine as being a great blood tonic. Those sensitive to oxalates may need to avoid beetroot to avoid digestive discomfort in the early stages of healing.

I had a friend over recently with an autistic son who because of his sensory issues was only up to smelling vegetables, rather than eating them. I offered her a taste of these beets and the beetroot kvass I had made. To our delight, this little boy and his younger brother were fighting over our food they enjoyed the taste so much.

Ingredients

- 3 beetroots
- 1 cinnamon stick and/or star anise
- 1 tsp orange zest
- 1 piece of turmeric
- 1 tsp sea salt
- ¼ tsp culture starter (if desired)

Making it

1. Chop beets in a food processor. Add the orange rind, cinnamon and grated turmeric to beets and mix together.
2. Place mix in a jar (about 500ml) and add sea salt or culture starter and pound with a wooden spoon to encourage the juices to release.
3. Cover with filtered water up to the shoulder (this allows for the food to expand as it ferments).
4. Leave on your kitchen bench top for four to seven days (depending on the heat of your kitchen). Keep in the fridge.

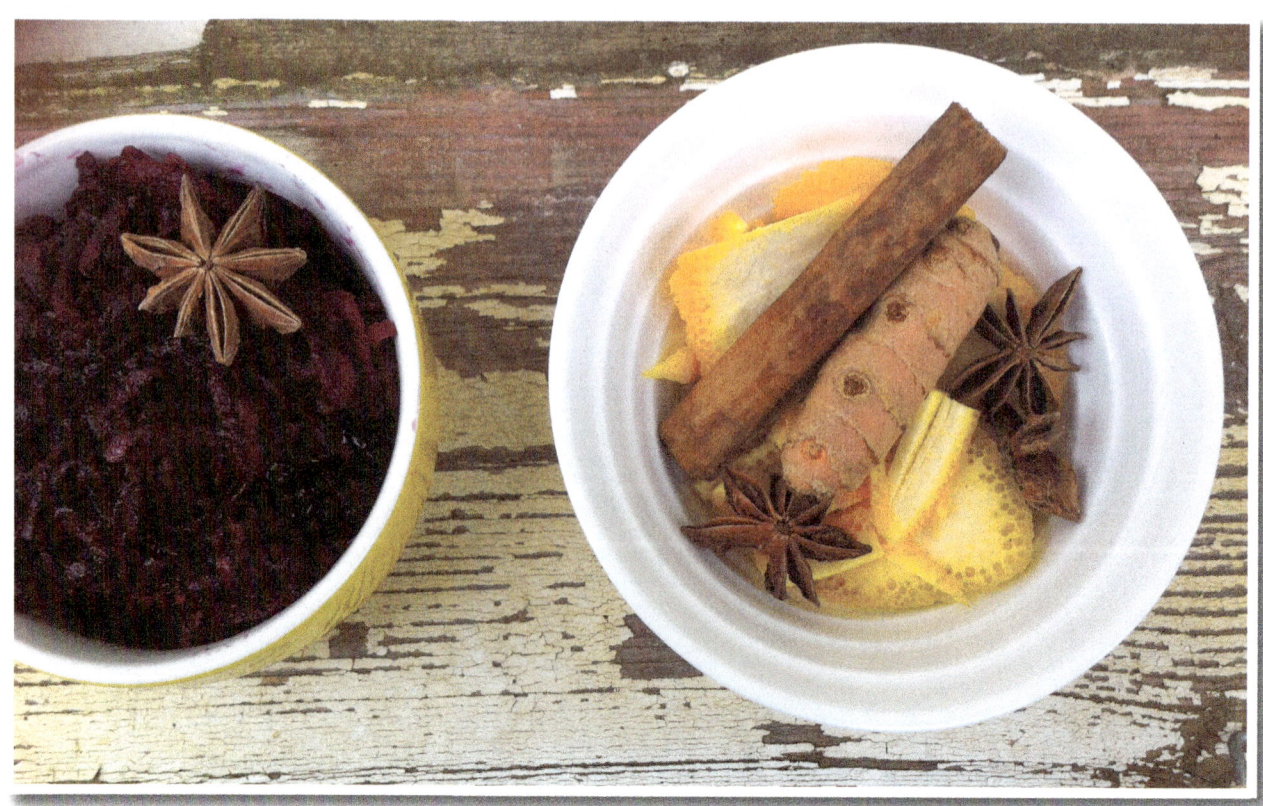

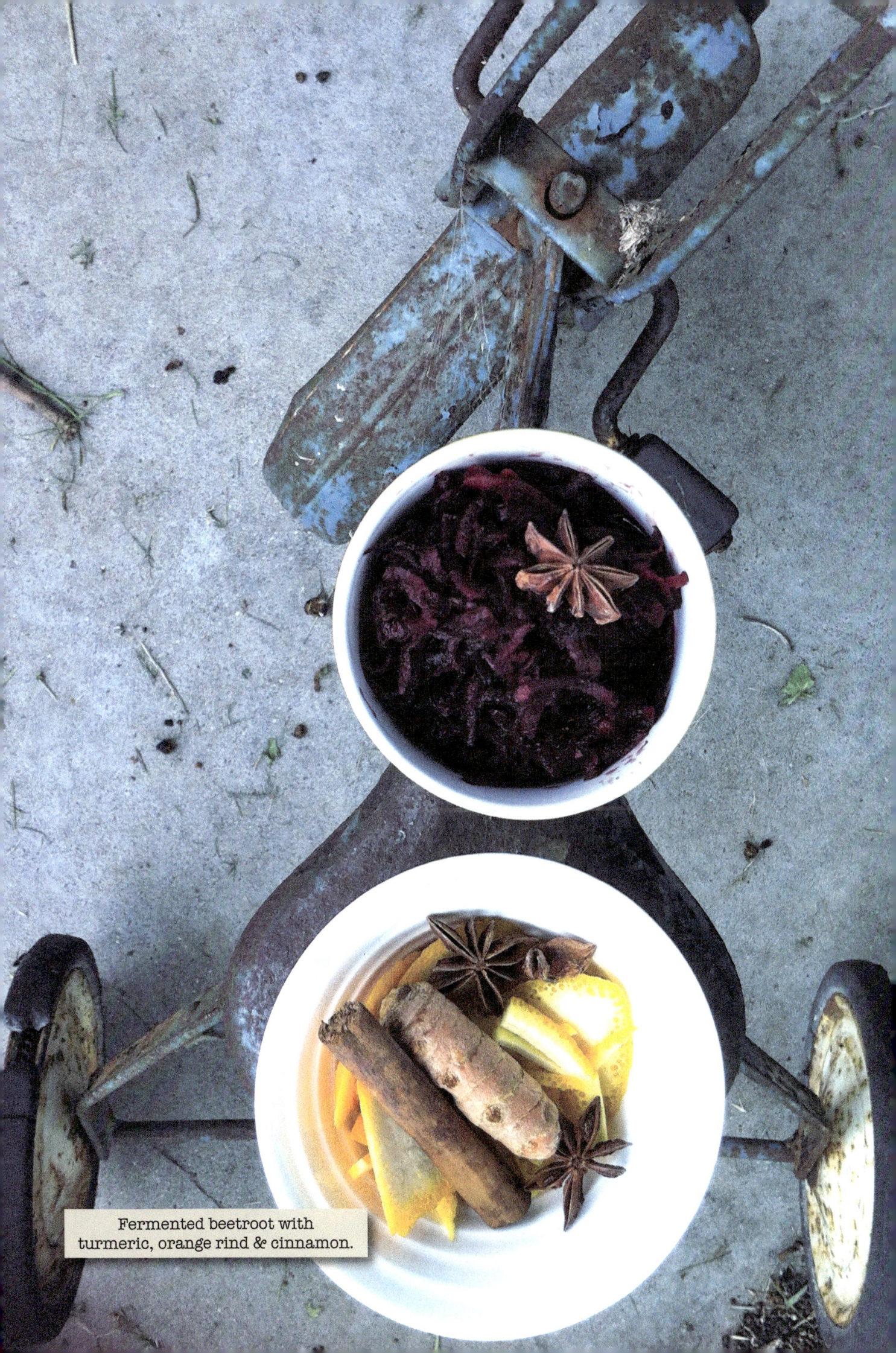

Fermented beetroot with turmeric, orange rind & cinnamon.

Dilly beans

Dilly beans are a lovely way for children to have a crunchy snack but still get the probiotic value from the food.

They are a great introduction to fermented foods for a lot of children. As I've mentioned, beetroot, beetroot kvass and pickled carrots are also fantastic starting points.

If you are still battling to get your children into probiotic vegetables, take heart. Bubbly, fruity probiotic drinks such as water kefir might be your way in.

Ingredients

- Handful of French beans (topped and tailed)
- 1 tsp Himalayan, Celtic or Macrobiotic salt
- Tsp Dill seeds
- Vine leaves
- 1 clove peeled garlic

Making it

1. Fill a 500 ml jar with organic green beans standing up, making sure you only pack to the shoulder of your vessel as they will expand with the fermentation process.
2. Add the garlic and two vine leaves (the leaves will help to keep them crunchy).
3. Add one teaspoon of sea salt.
4. Cover with filtered water.
5. Let the jar sit on your kitchen counter out of direct sunlight for four to five days.
6. Keep them in the fridge for four to five days before trying them as they will get better with time.

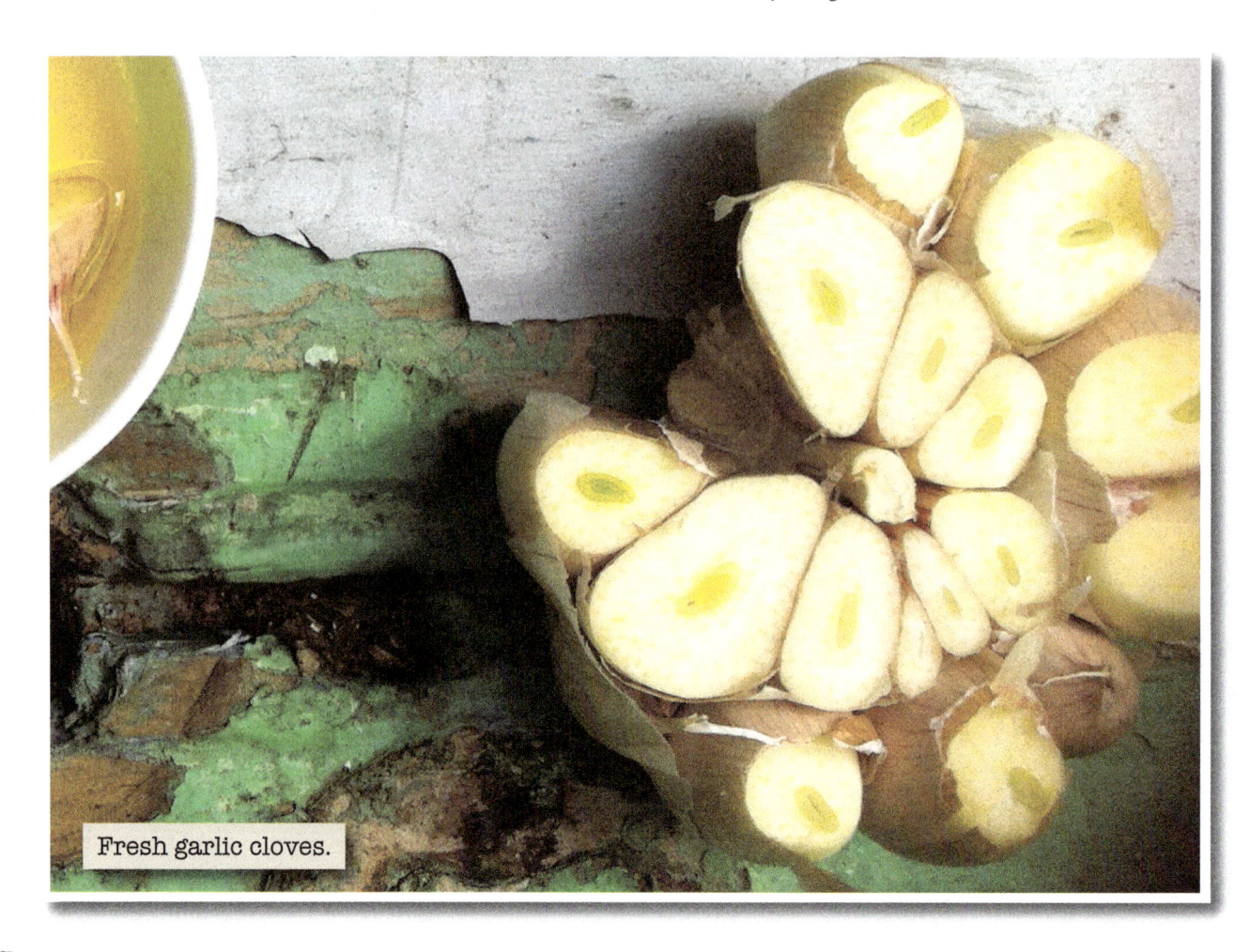

Fresh garlic cloves.

Dilly beans.

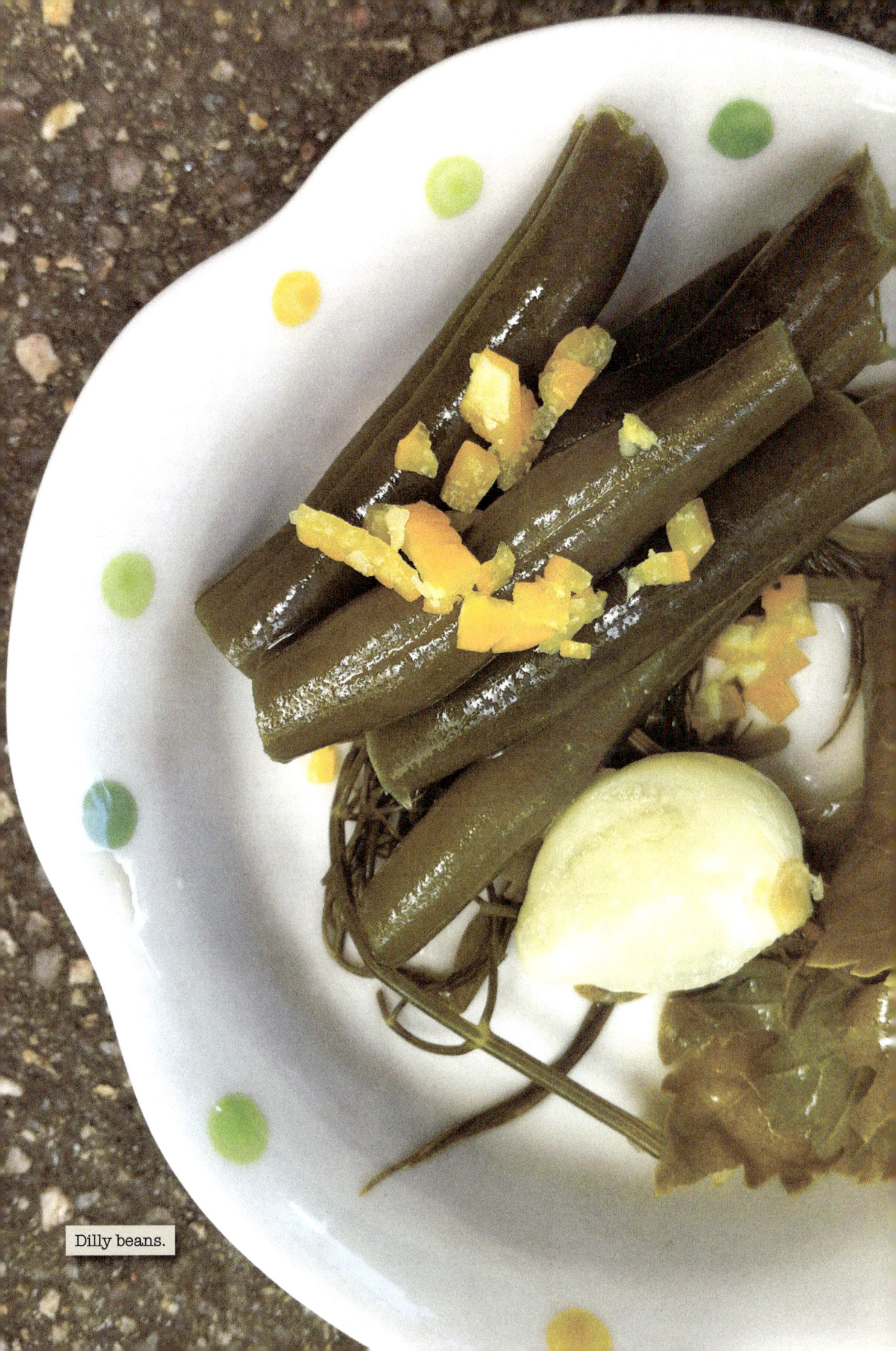

Kimchi

This Korean staple is fantastic for those who love that extra kick of ginger and chilli.

In most cultures around the world, fermented food is a feature. The Japanese have miso soup, the Russians have sauerkraut, even our own tomato sauce would have been preserved in salt in years gone by. I wonder what our nation's general health would be like if fermented foods were reintroduced. Would we see less obesity, less heart disease, less food sensitivity? There are many researchers looking into these very subjects. I am hopeful we as a society will continue to embrace this knowledge and begin to reclaim our power over our health. I hope that we can really make the connection between food and medicine and live by that old axiom: 'You are what you eat'.

> This kimchi recipe is really for the adults. It's a staple Korean food that has made its way into the hearts and tummies of people the world over. There are many variations, I hope you enjoy this one.

Ingredients

- 1 green cabbage
- 3 carrots
- 1 daikon radish
- 1 tbs grated ginger
- 3 garlic cloves chopped finely
- ½ tsp dried chili flakes
- 1 tablespoon sea salt

Making it

Take outer leaves off your cabbage and reserve the cleanest one for later. Cut the head into quarters and remove the core.

1. Finely chop using a food processor if you have one.
2. Put cabbage in a large bowl, and toss with 2 tsp sea salt. Let sit at room temperature for ten minutes.
3. Using a thick wooden spoon, pound the cabbage for about five minutes to help release the natural juices. Put into your sterilised (1lt) glass jar.
4. Layer cabbage with carrot and then daikon – adding your ginger, garlic and chili as you go along. Pack the vegetables in the jar nice and tight but only to the shoulder.
5. Make additional brine water to top up jar until it covers the veggies. To do this, dissolve 1 tsp salt into two cups room temperature filtered water.
6. Pour this into the jars until the cabbage is covered.
7. Fold up your outside cabbage leaf and put it on top of your veggies to weight them down. You don't want them to come above the water.
8. Close your lid, wrap it up so it doesn't get into any direct sunlight and give it ten days.
9. After this time, take the top leaf off and any darkened veggies.

Kimchi gets better as it matures in the fridge. Will keep for many months.

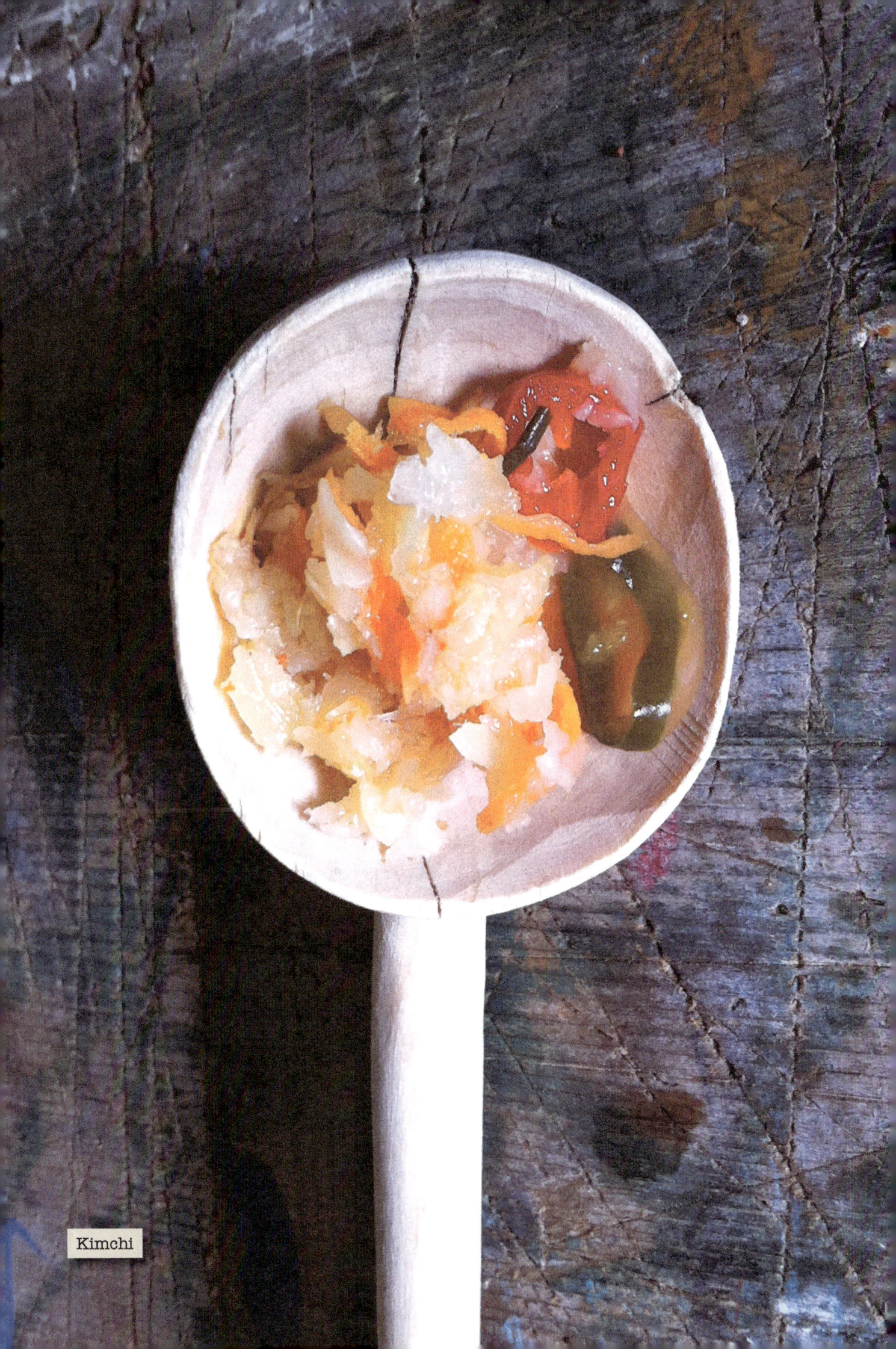

Kimchi

Lacto fermented tomato salsa

Organic tomato, Spanish onion, garlic from the garden and lemons from a friend.

This is a very easy mix. No real recipe is needed, just a knowledge of what goes well with what. The general rule I like to follow is if it goes well together in a salad, chances are it will go well together in a jar.

This salsa would also be great with some red or green capsicum and chilli.

Ingredients

- 1 tsp of salt
- 1 punnet organic cherry tomatoes halved
- 1 Spanish onion finely sliced
- 2 cloves of garlic chopped
- 1/2 tsp of lemon zested, basil leaf or oregano
- ¼ tsp culture starter

Making it

1. To a 500ml jar add a quarter of a teaspoon of culture starter and a teaspoon of salt (culture starter is particularly helpful when using fruits).
2. Add veggies and top with filtered water. Leave on your kitchen counter out of direct sunlight for three days.
3. It will get better after you put it in the fridge for a few days more.

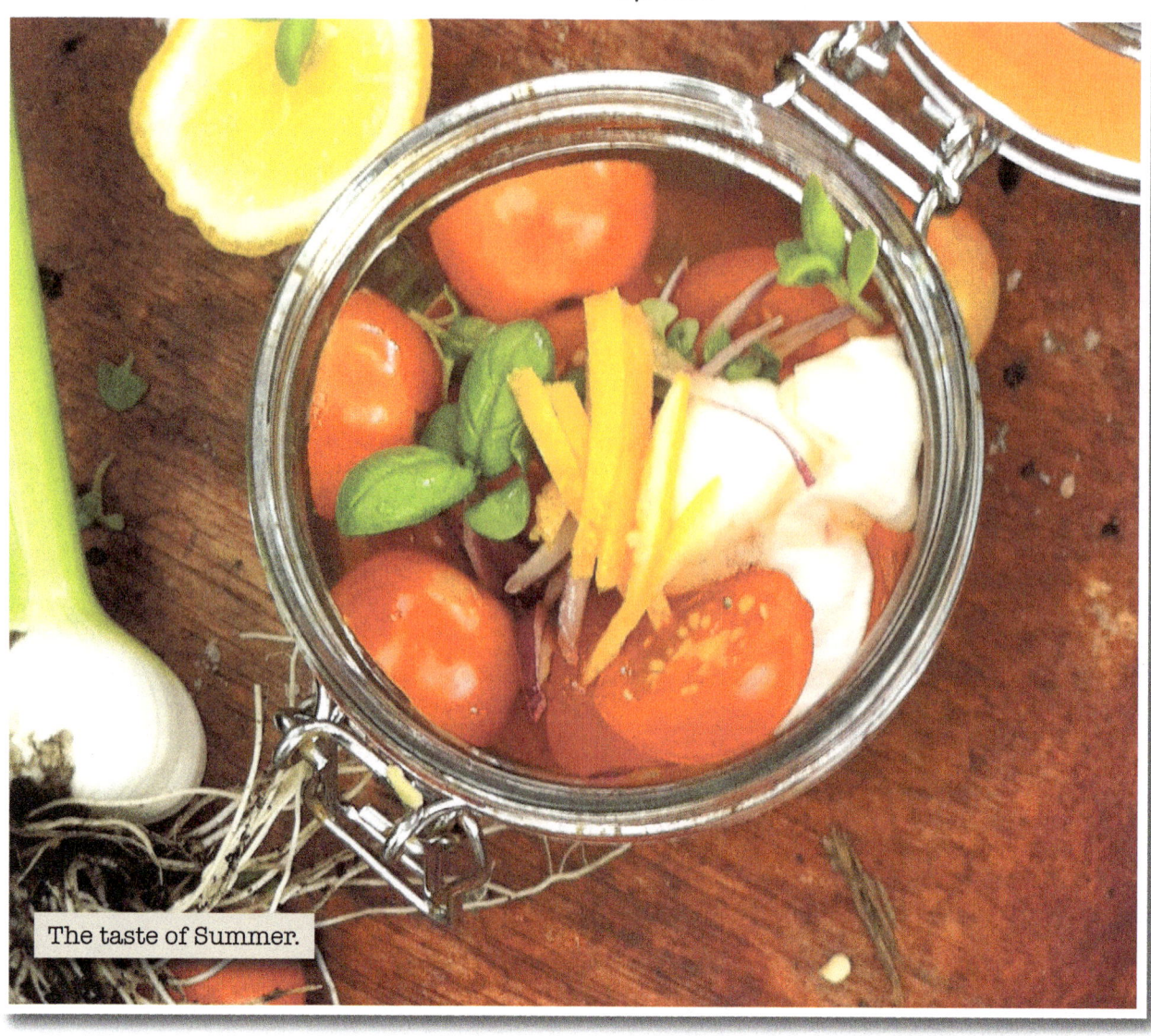

The taste of Summer.

Sides & Snacks

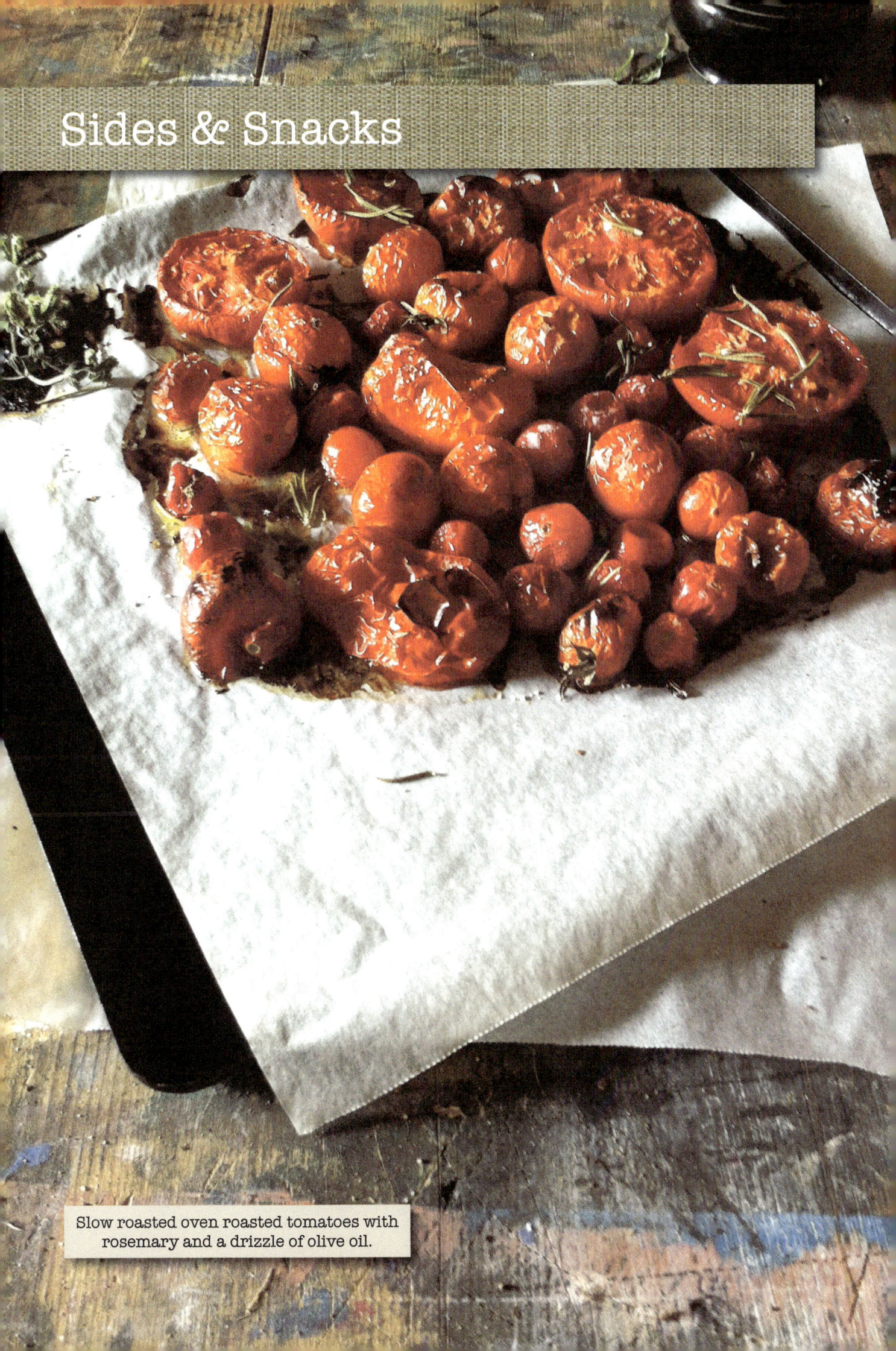

Slow roasted oven roasted tomatoes with rosemary and a drizzle of olive oil.

Chicken liver pate

Lemon thyme chicken liver pate: It's hard to believe this stuff is medicine, however organ meats are one of life's forgotten treasures.

Most people remember the horror of being served a piece of liver as a child and feeling pretty traumatised by the gritty, cloying texture. Some people never get over it.

All I can say is that I tried to avoid that with my children and by whizzing this up with a good amount of ghee and cultured cream - it is now my oldest daughter's favourite.

Liver is an easy way for the body to get access to Vitamin A and iron. If the gut isn't functioning, as it should, no amount of carrots are going to cut it, you simply won't be able to absorb their nutrients.

Note: I would only ever eat organic liver. I order it through our local health food store and then make a good-sized batch so we can have just a tiny amount every day.

Ingredients

- 100 grams of liver
- Two shallots, chopped
- ½ cup of ghee/butter or olive oil and 1 tbs for frying shallots
- 2 tbs lemon thyme leaves
- Salt to taste
- 50gms softened butter (to help seal the pate)

Making it

1. Wash livers and take out all the connective tissue.
2. Leave livers to soak with the juice of half a lemon and cover with some water for a few hours. This removes the bitter taste.
3. Strain and rinse livers with fresh water. Pat dry with kitchen paper. Fry shallots in a little butter till soft but not brown.
4. Add liver and lemon thyme and fry until brown but still a bit pink on the inside.
5. Allow to cool slightly. Whizz up in food processor until very smooth and adding the remaining ghee, butter or coconut oil if you need to be dairy free. Do this slowly, tasting as you go. Add a sprinkle of salt so it is to your liking.
6. Pour into individual ramekins. Wait till cool and pour some extra melted butter, ghee or coconut oil on top to seal.
7. I store these in sandwich bags in the fridge.

Chicken Liver Pate.

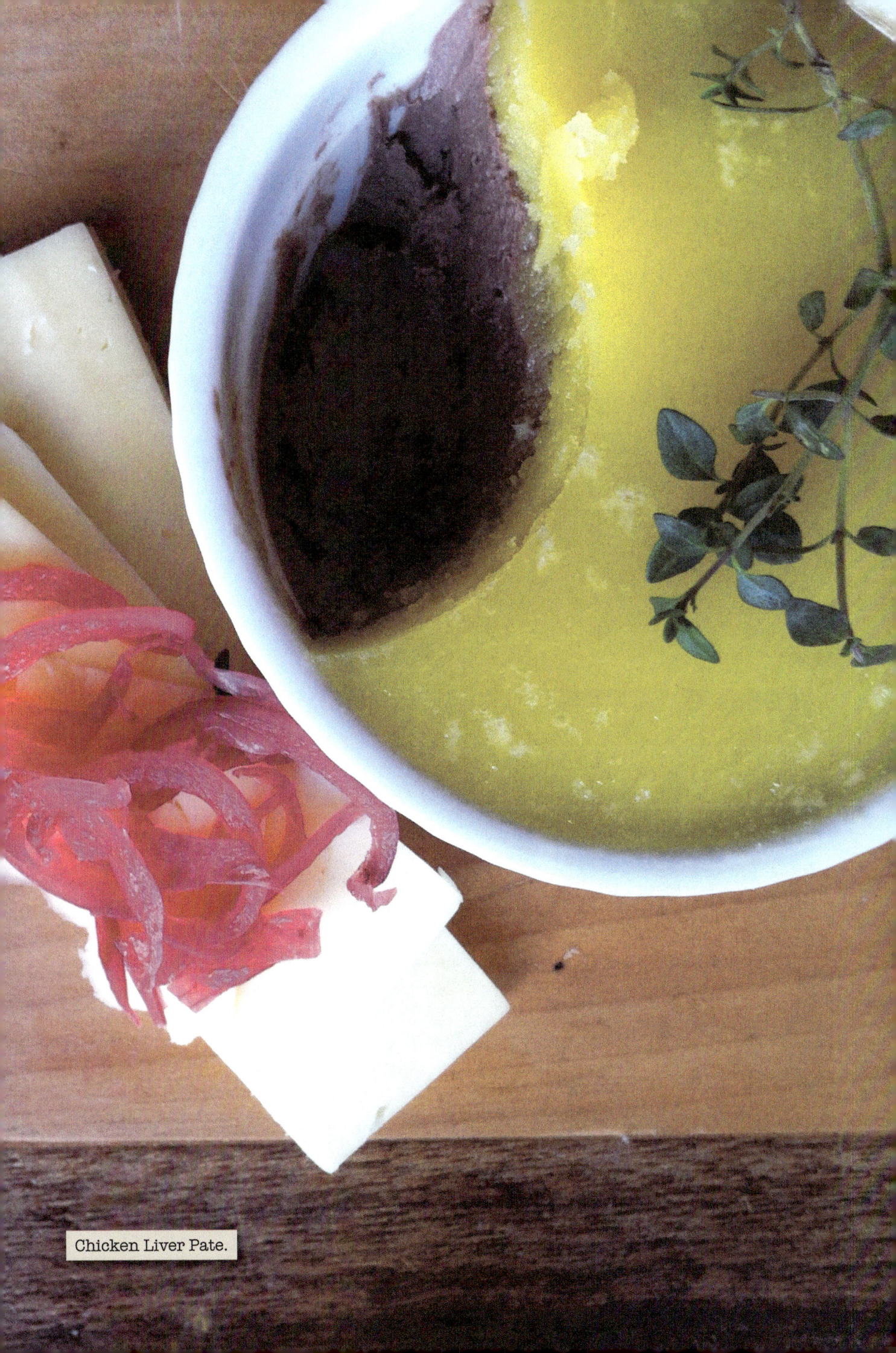

Slow roasted brussels sprouts with butter & rosemary

Brussels sprouts are an ick food for lots of people - especially children.

I find they taste totally different when you par boil and roast them slowly with butter/coconut oil, bringing out their natural sweetness.

They are loaded with Vitamin A, C, potassium and calcium.

Fry up some organic bacon or have them with lamb meatballs and a yoghurt dip.

Ingredients

- 12 Brussels sprouts
- 1 large rasher of bacon
- 1 tsp chopped dried rosemary
- Butter to taste

Making it

1. Halve each Brussels sprout with a sharp knife
2. Par boil on the stove top
3. Drain and put in a baking dish with butter, duck fat or tallow and bake at 180 degrees C for about 30-40 mins
4. Fry bacon on the stove top until crispy and chop into small pieces
5. Bring the Brussels and bacon together, scatter with rosemary, toss with butter and add salt to taste.

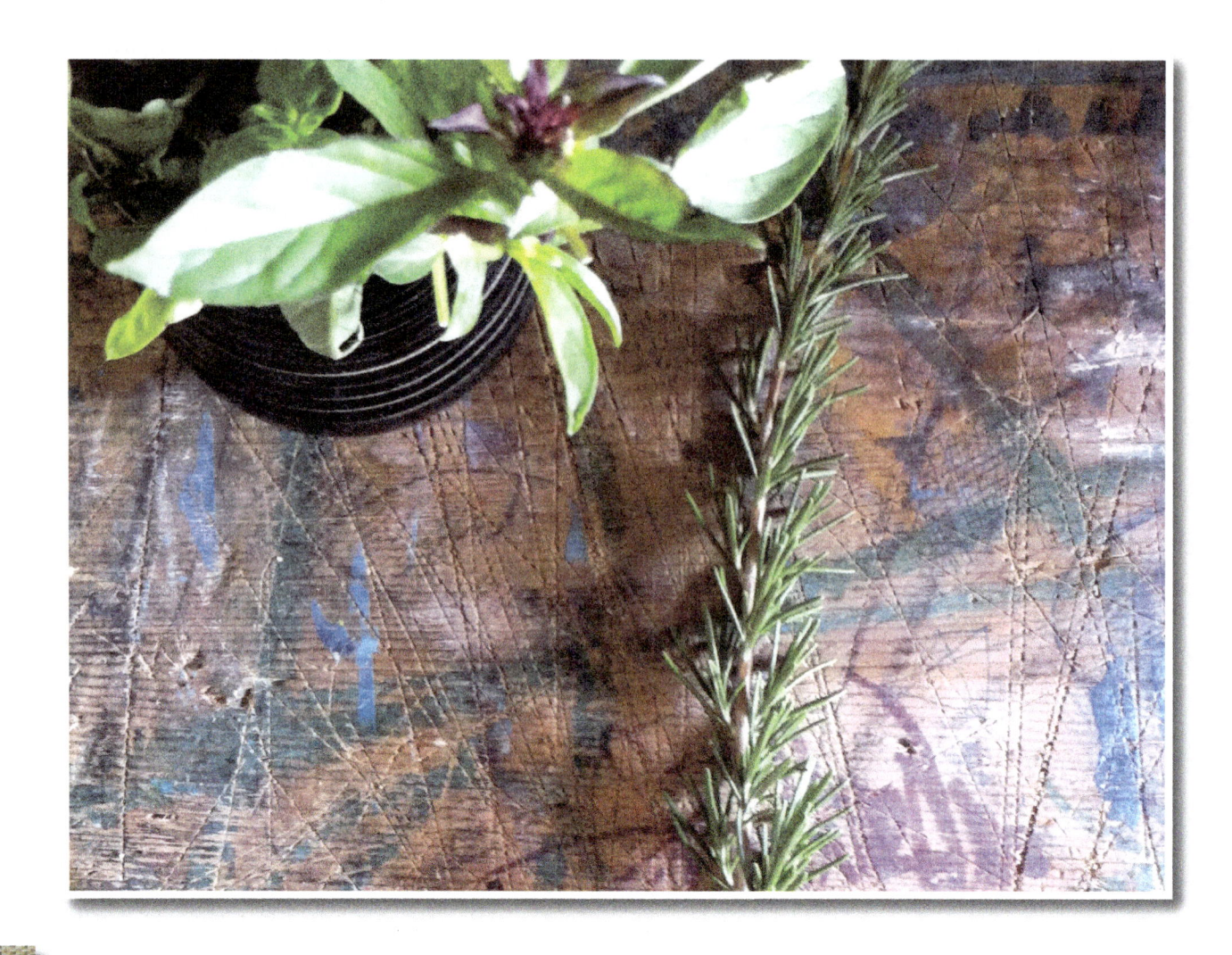

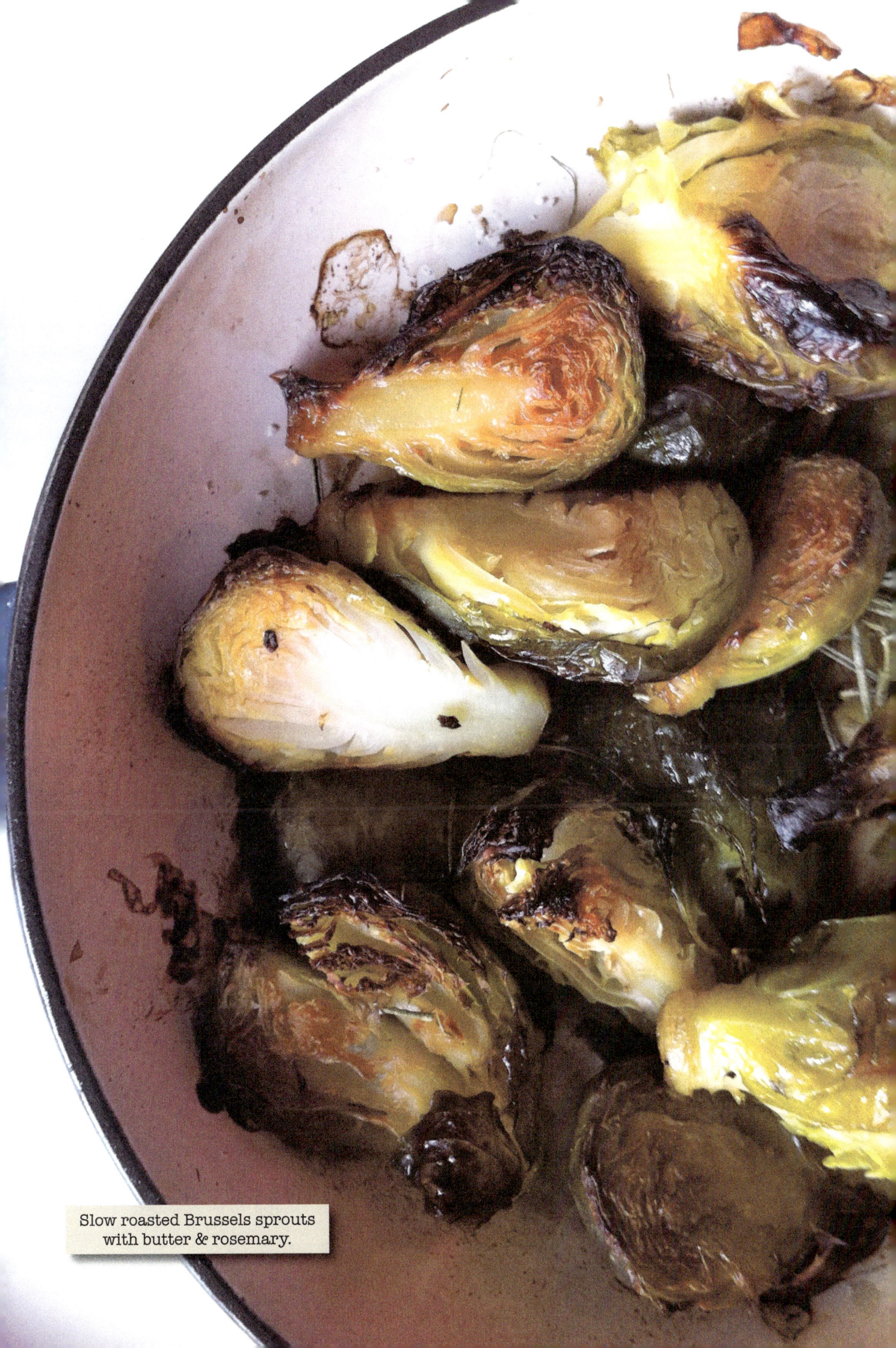

Slow roasted Brussels sprouts with butter & rosemary.

Gut healing jelly cups

I created these delicious little things on a day when we were heading for a top of 40 degrees.

I wanted minimal stove time.

The windows were closed, the curtains were drawn. We were ready for the onslaught. All we needed now was a quick, no-fuss breakfast.

Plums from my Dad's garden. Deep purple skin, plump, incredibly juicy.

Spray-free blueberries from our local grower, mixed with banana and avocado.

Homemade yoghurt, organic mango, toasted sunflower seeds.

These were devoured.

Note: We use red Great Lakes Gelatin to make jelly (but you could use any high quality gelatine derived from grass fed cows). As mentioned, gelatine is touted as having incredible gut healing qualities.

It is very high in collagen, so I like to think of it as a natural beauty product - as all healthy food is really.

Ingredients

- 5 plums
- 4 tsp gelatine
- 1 cup blueberries
- ¼ ripe banana
- ¼ ripe avocado
- 1 cup yoghurt
- Toasted sunflower seeds (soaked and sprouted is best)

Making it

Jelly

1. Take about five plums and two cups of filtered water. Bring to the boil and let simmer till you get a lovely deep pink colour from the fruit.
2. Strain fruit with a sieve, put warm liquid back into saucepan and quickly stir in the Great Lakes gelatin (I get the red one online).
3. Pour the jelly into whatever glasses or paper cups you plan to serve in and allow to firm up in the freezer. This should take about half an hour. Max.
4. In the meantime, blend a cup of frozen blueberries with a quarter of a ripe banana and a quarter of a ripe avocado using a stick mixer. You could use any combination of fruit for this but a little avocado gives you a creamy consistency, the banana some sweetness - you could even add a tsp of good quality cocoa and raw honey if you really need a chocolate fix.
5. When the jelly is firm, bring your glasses back to the bench and spoon the blueberry mix on top and allow the mix to settle for a minute.

If the berries are frozen they will be a nice stable table for the yoghurt which is to follow.

I had some pre-made 24 hour yoghurt which I gently spooned on the top. If you use a tall glass, it will be easier to get the layering effect.

If you needed a dairy free option, Substitute with coconut cream. If yoghurt or coconut cream are not an option you could try some cultured cream.

I then added some sliced fruit. We had mango at home but passionfruit, more blueberries, mixed berries, any kind of ripe, seasonal fruit would be delicious.

We topped with toasted sunflower seeds because we are slowly bringing nuts back into the diet after severe allergy - plus it's nice to have a nut free option if you need it.

You could also go heavier on the nuts and seeds and do a whole layer, try a mix of sunflower, pumpkin, walnuts, almonds...

Or you could just toast some fresh coconut and sprinkle on top.

Gut healing jelly cups.

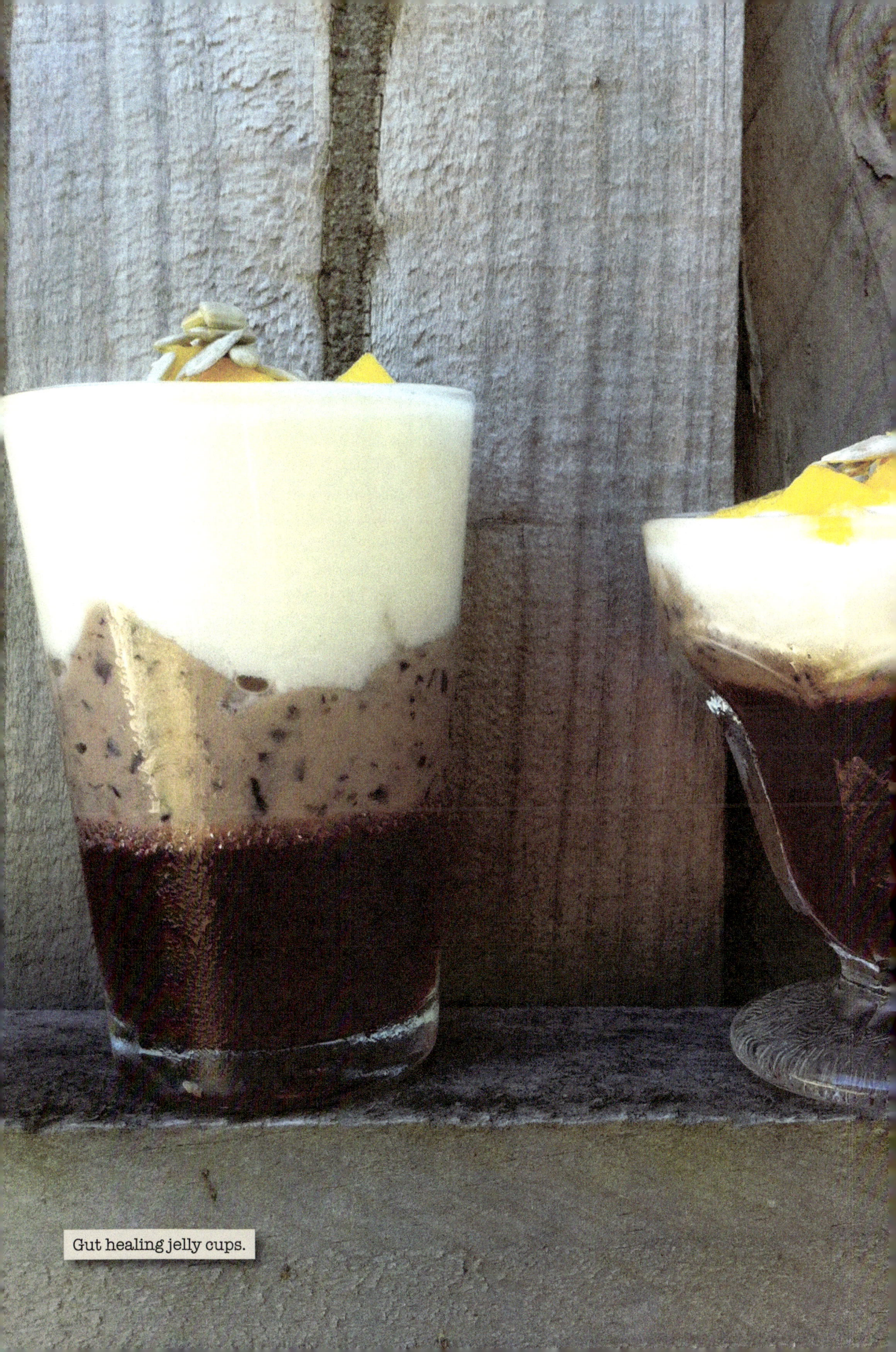

Boiled egg on salmon

Who says you need toast to have an egg for brekky?

I admit, I love to dip a good bit of sourdough into a soft-boiled egg but I also like to know that I can still enjoy without.

They are a massive source of nutrition. For perfect soft-boiled eggs every time, I put eggs into a small saucepan full of cold water.

When the water starts to boil, I set my timer for two minutes. When the two minutes is up, I submerge the egg in cold water. This way they are soft and gooey every time, without fail.

Serve with wild caught salmon, fresh barramundi and mushy peas or avocado and sauerkraut.

For a long time, even the sight of eggs made me shudder.

With my oldest daughter being anaphylactic to them, I did everything I could to avoid them.

Other brekky options we do at home are:

- Poached eggs with bacon, avocado, mushrooms, roasted tomato and spinach
- Cheese souffles with asparagus
- Berry mousse
- Pumpkin custards
- Banana custards
- Pumpkin soup
- Chicken soup
- Meatballs of any kind
- Turkish brekky with boiled eggs, sliced cucumbers, tomato and tasty cheese
- Brekky jelly cups
- Apple or pear crumble
- Avocado, banana, berry, coconut smoothie
- Yoghurt with pepitas, walnuts, dried apricots and sliced banana
- Chia pudding
- Sticky pork chops with broccoli

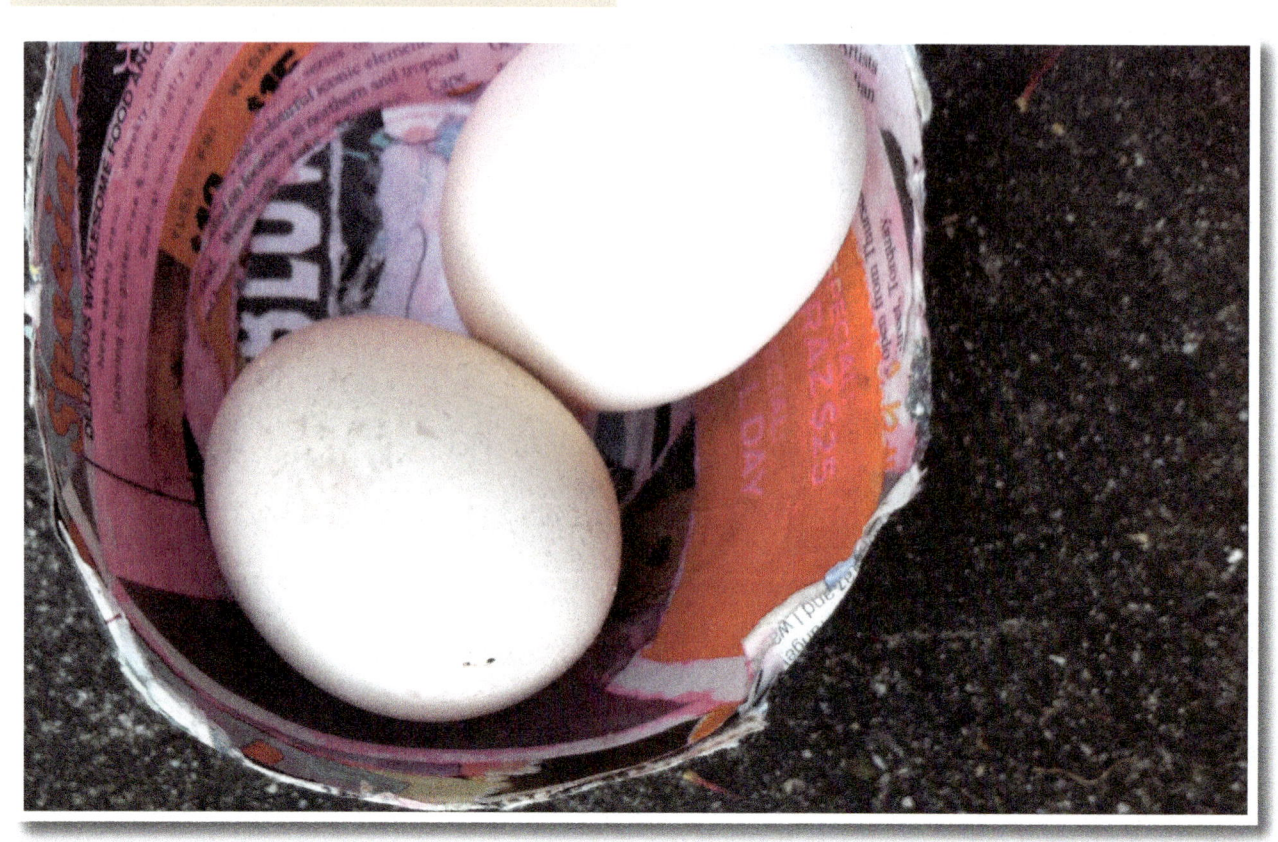

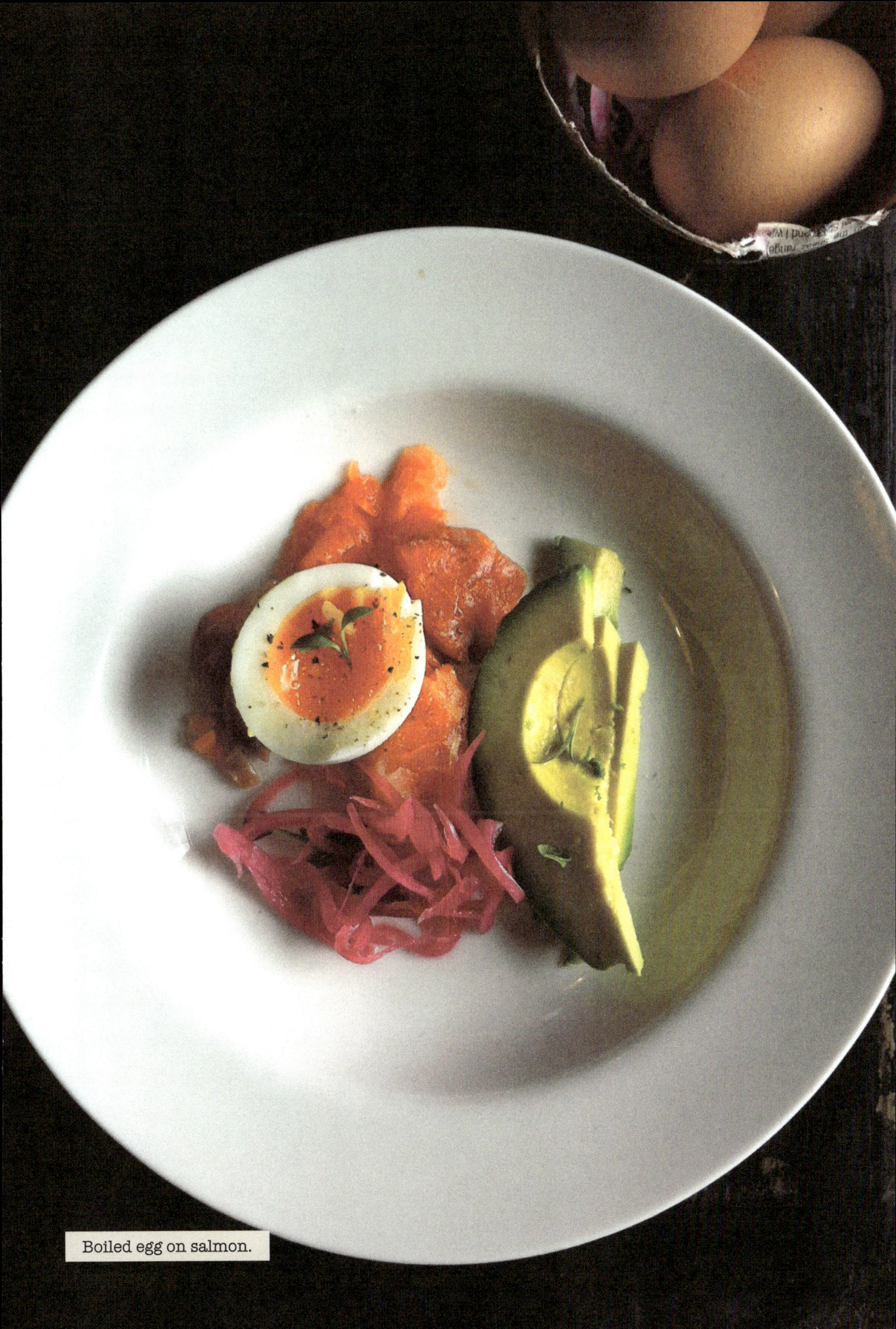

Boiled egg on salmon.

Spiced beetroot carpaccio

A very easy salad. Gently boil beetroot with skins on for about an hour with the lid on. Be careful not to nick or chop tails to keep the deep purple colour.

Add one star anise, a tsp of orange peel and a cinnamon quill if you can handle spice. When tender, gently rub the skins off with your fingers.

Slice thinly and dress with organic lemon peel, garlic infused olive oil, flavoured salt and micro greens (we used coriander this time).

Serve with lamb chops and rosemary yoghurt. Add finely chopped lemon peel on top for garnish.

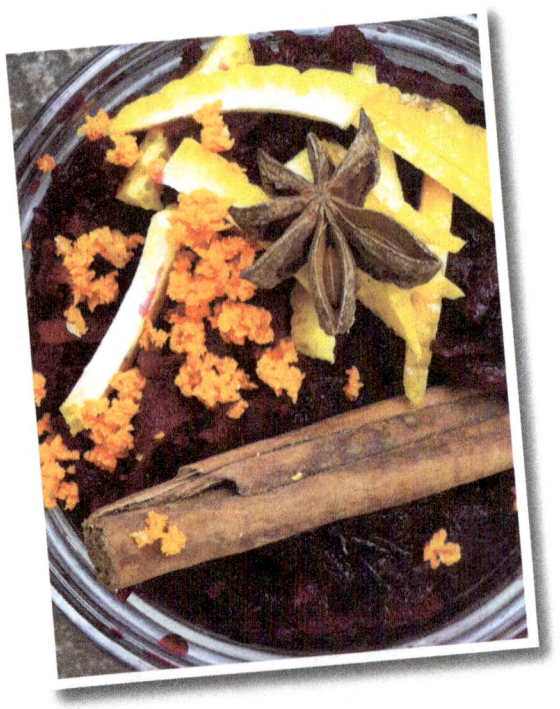

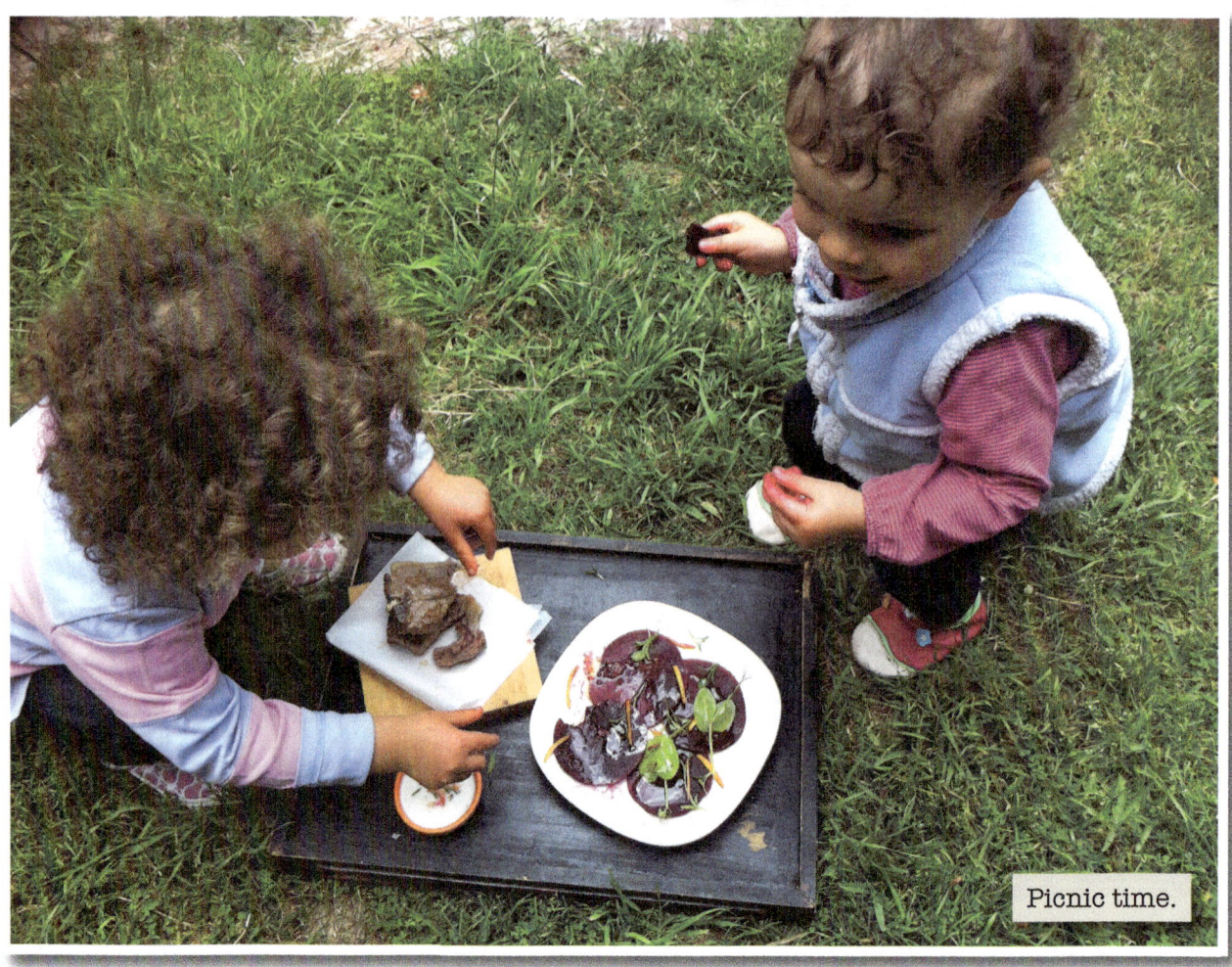

Picnic time.

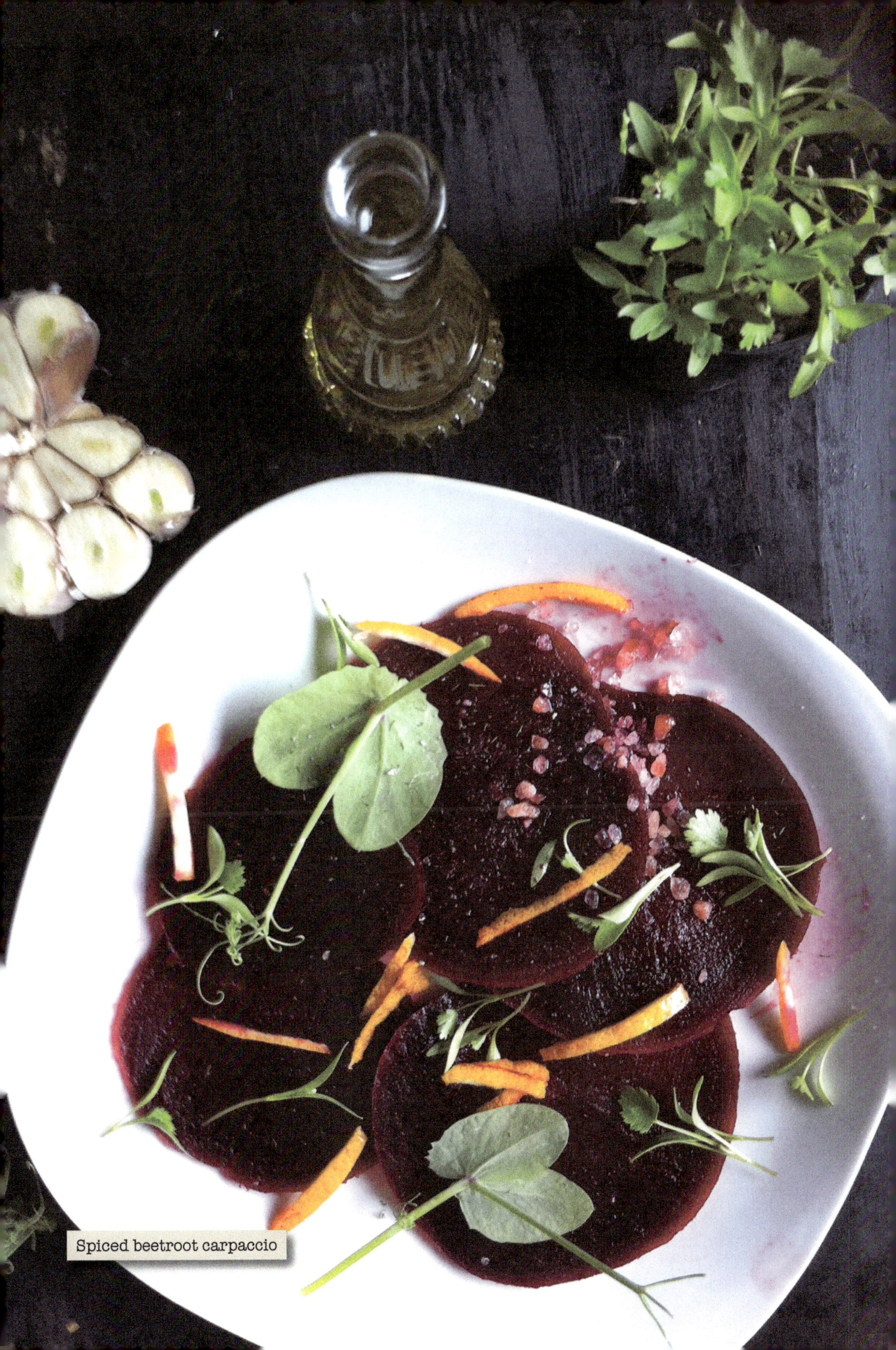

Spiced beetroot carpaccio

Fried mushrooms with thyme

These are a great side or a stand alone snack.

Fry up approximately 10 button mushrooms with lashings of butter, ghee or coconut oil until soft.

Add three sprigs of thyme and finish with a sprinkle of salt and cultured cream.

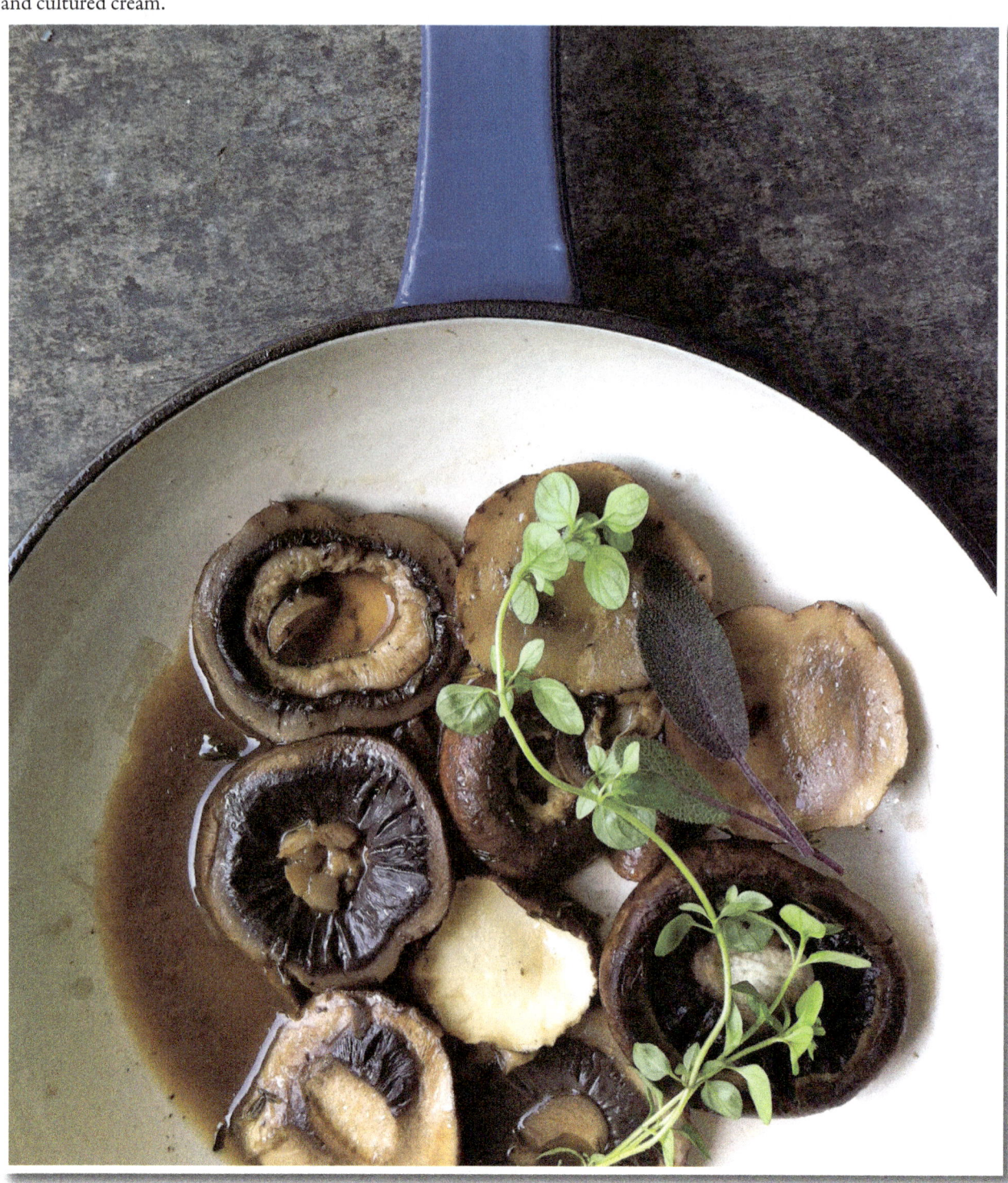

Soups

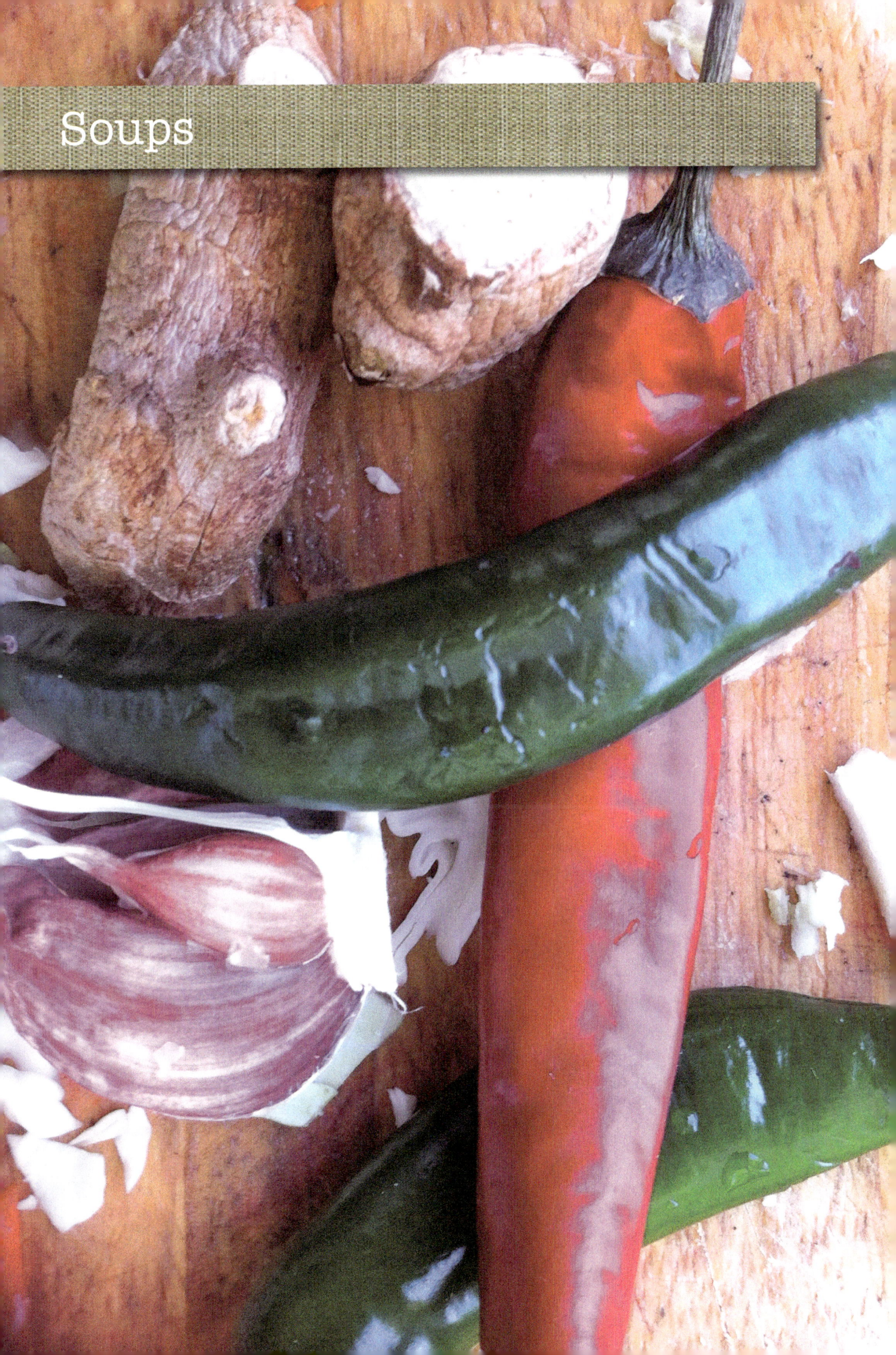

Borscht

Another great way to get my children to drink chicken broth on country Victorian days that are rainy then sunny, then rainy again.

Ingredients

- 4 beets
- 2 cloves garlic
- 2 carrots
- 1 half small cabbage
- 6 cups chicken stock, or water
- 1 leek, onion or shallot
- Apple cider vinegar (1 tsp to serve)
- A sprig of dill
- Yoghurt or cultured cream to serve
- Pinch of salt

Making it

1. In a large (preferably stainless steel) pot, add finely chopped leek, onion, garlic and fry in butter or ghee.
2. When softened add beets and carrots cut into small cubes.
3. Add, finely chopped cabbage, stock, a pinch of salt and allow to simmer with the lid partially on for about one hour.
4. Serve in bowls and add 1 tsp of apple cider vinegar (into warm but not boiling hot soup).
5. Top with cultured cream or yoghurt and chopped dill.
6. I also do one final slug of the best olive oil I have.

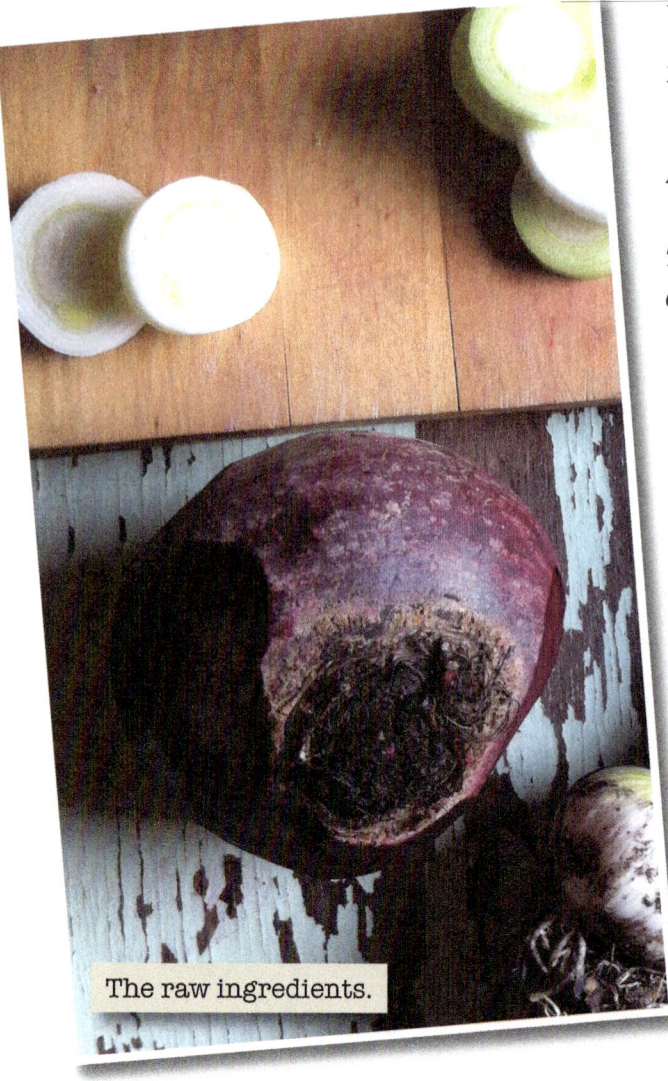

The raw ingredients.

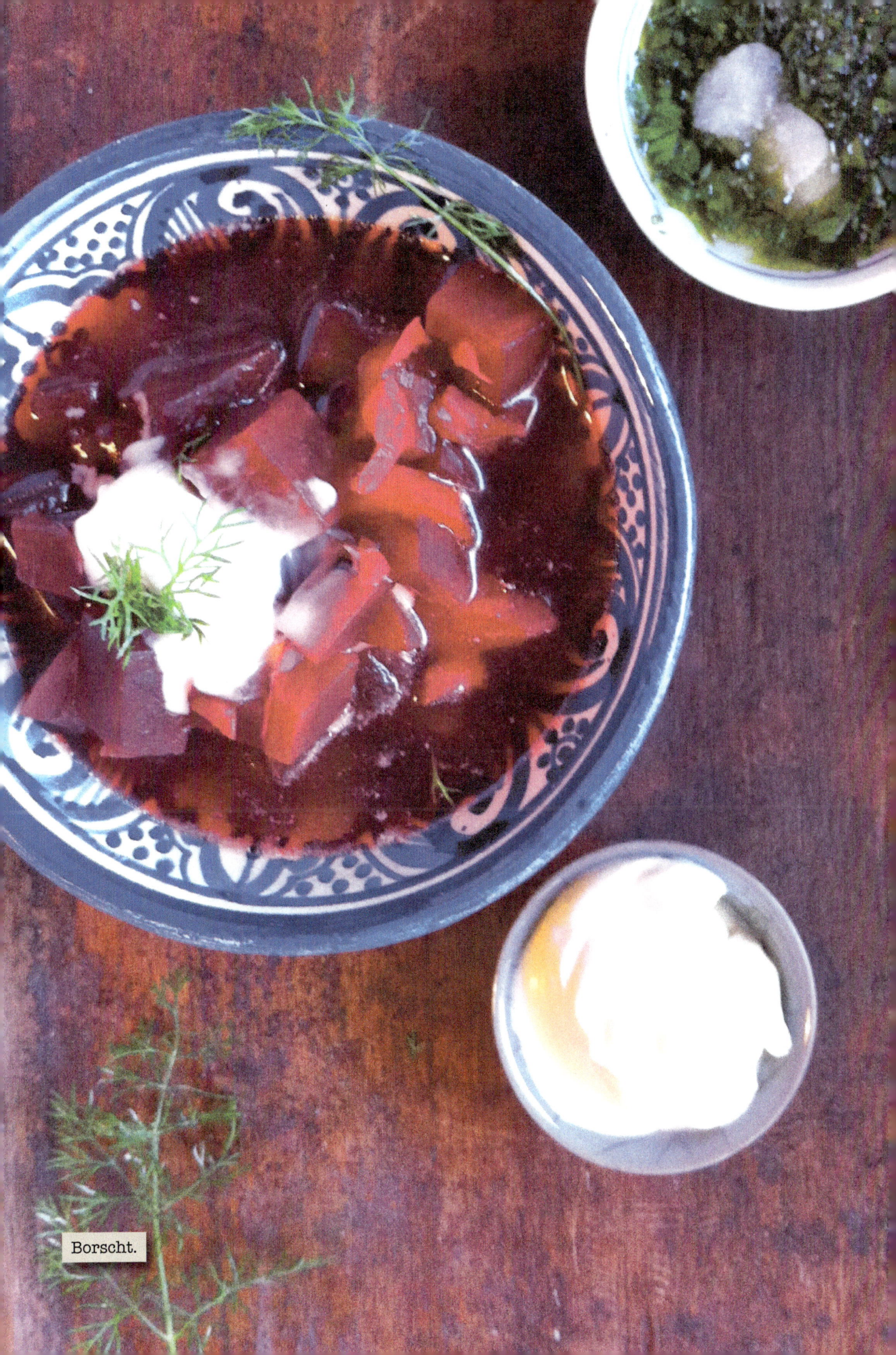

Borscht.

excellent

The easiest pumpkin soup ever

It's a simple soup. Thick, sweet and a great way to get my kids to drink meat stock which is rich in gut healing properties glycine and collagen.

The problem is, I hate peeling the skin of the pumpkin.

To avoid this, I've taken to splitting a few butternut pumpkins down the middle and turning it face down to roast in the oven at 180 degrees C for about 40 minutes with a few garlic cloves in their skin.

In the meantime, I fry a leek, four garlic cloves and two sage leaves in a saucepan until soft. Do taste at this point. It really must be soft otherwise you'll have chunks of onion to chew on.

Butter or ghee is nice for frying. Add coconut oil if you want another healing food in the mix.

> You could even add coconut milk and lemon grass if you want a more Asian flavour.

When the pumpkin is completely soft, I peel off the skin and add a litre or two of chicken broth (I always have broth or stock on the go).

Add just enough to almost cover your pumpkin and whizz up with a stick mixer. Add more broth if you want a thinner consistency.

Warm through, add salt to taste and a dash of yoghurt or cultured cream.

Pack away the remaining roast pumpkin and use in quick and easy chicken salads or turn into a dip.

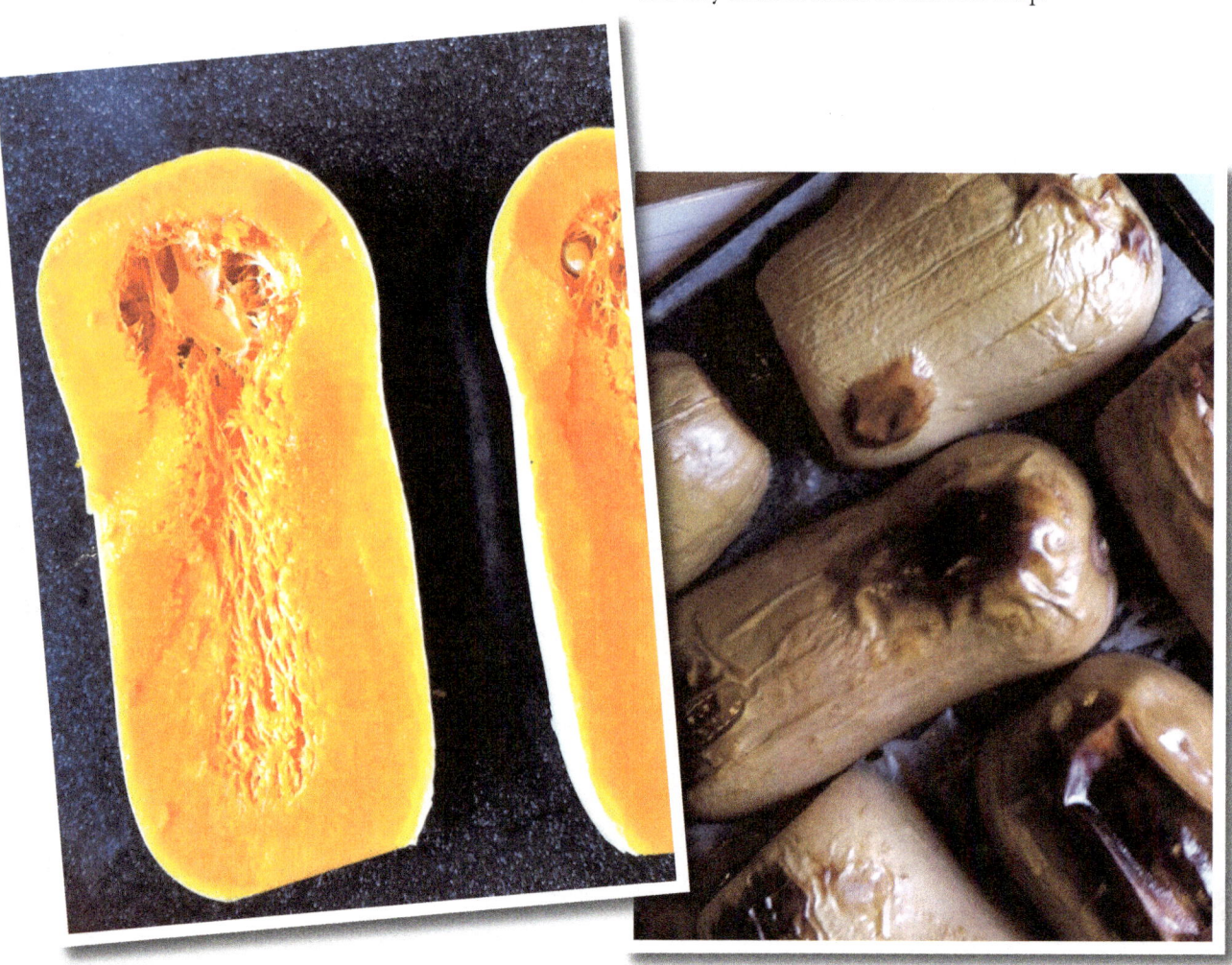

The easiest pumpkin soup ever

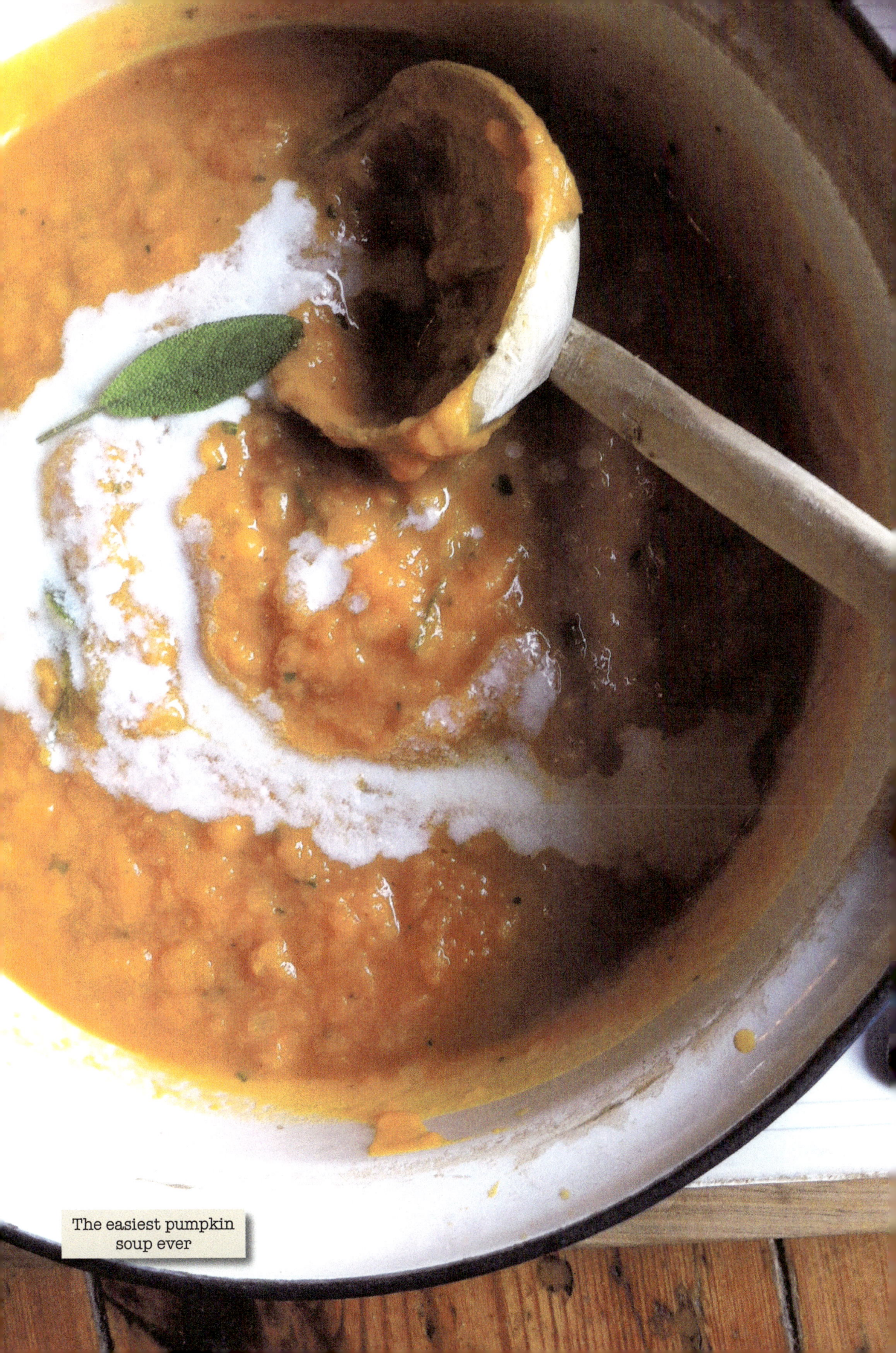

Cauliflower & leek soup

This was very yummy. Three-year-old loved it. 17-month-old did not like at all.

During this time, we've been very lucky to not have to deal with too much picky eating.

I have always offered a variety of flavours and asked our girls to try things.

I never made a fuss when or if the food was rejected, however, I remembered well the advice a dietitian gave me which was: "It's your job as a mum to decide what and when and the child's job to decide if and how much."

We are very fortunate that this general rule worked pretty well.

Ingredients

- One small head of cauliflower (preferably cut into florets and roasted, I often don't have time and it's still very nice.)
- 1 large leek
- 3 cloves of garlic
- 1 large shallot
- 6 cups chicken stock, or water
- Pinch of salt
- A sprig of thyme
- Celery leaves or stalks

Making it

1. Fry leek, garlic, shallot in butter/ghee/duck fat/or coconut oil until soft.
2. Add cauliflower florets, thyme and celery stalks (not chopped if you have severe tummy problems) and take out celery whole at the end.
3. Just cover with chicken stock and filtered water (home made only).
4. Bring to the boil and simmer for about 40 minutes.
5. Take out celery and thyme.
6. Whizz with a stick blender.
7. Serve with cultured cream or homemade yoghurt and sauerkraut on top.

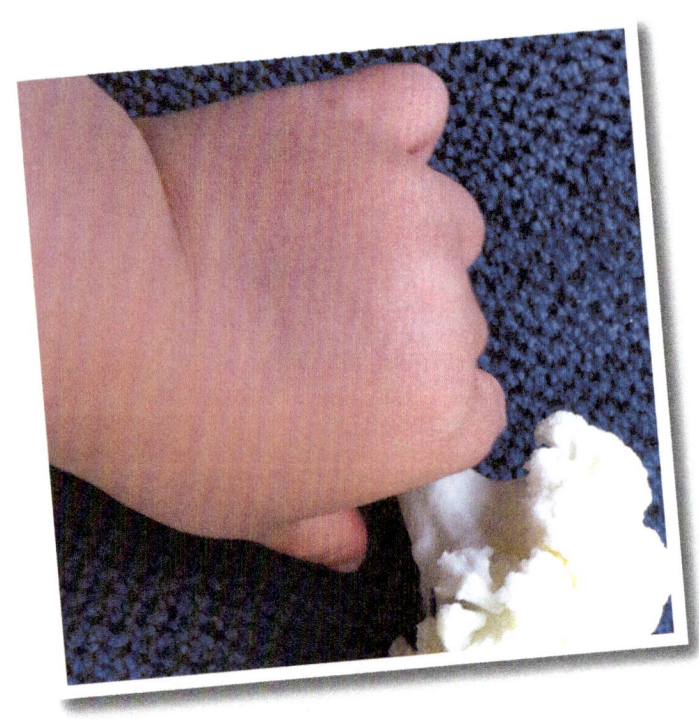

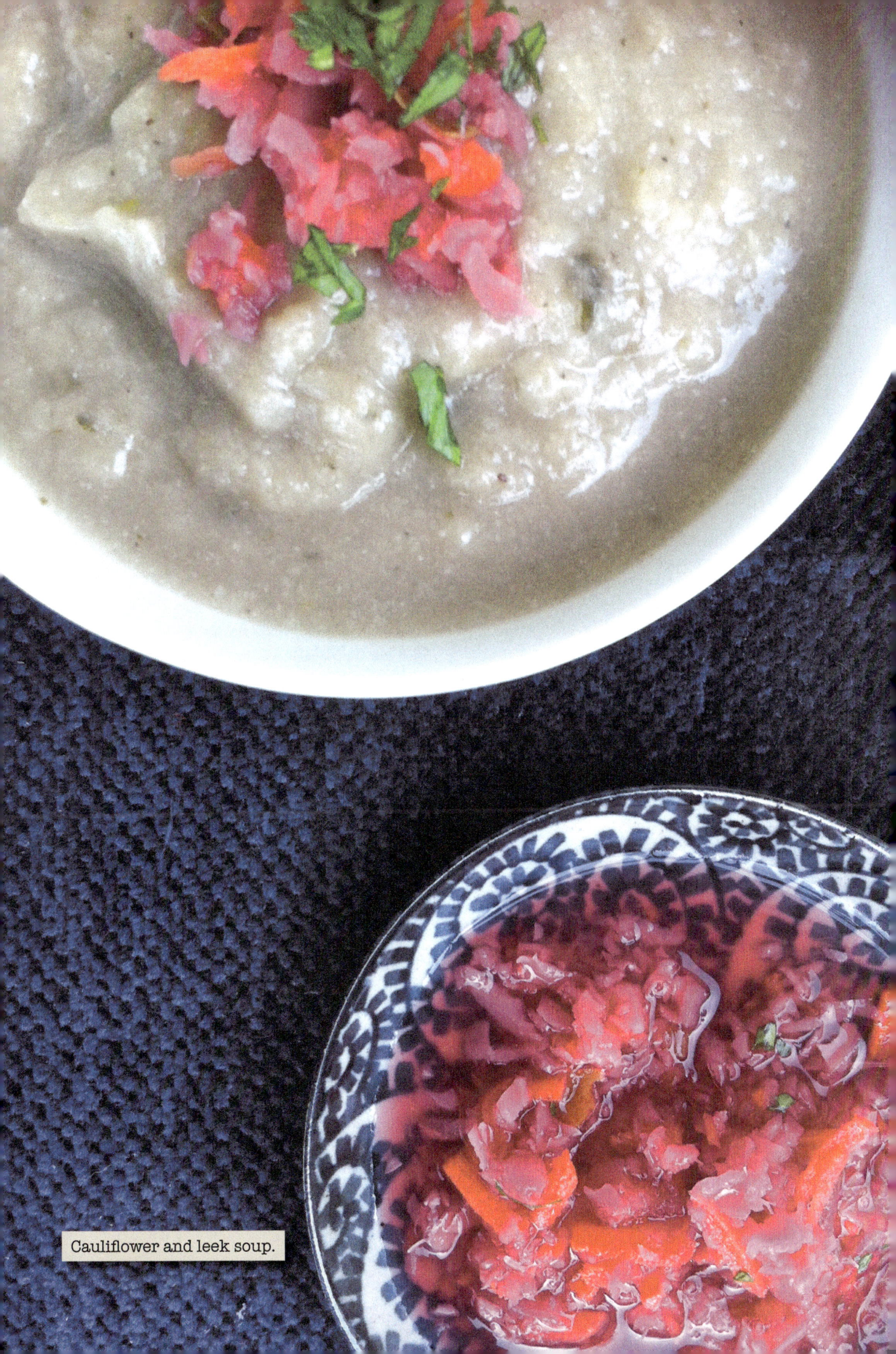

Cauliflower and leek soup.

Greek-style chicken soup

This is one of my favourite soups ever. Known as avgolemono, the traditional flavours in this beautiful Greek soup are something I remember from my childhood very well.

Normally served with rice, I have omitted this for now. The GAPS Diet essentially cuts out all grains and heavily starchy foods for a temporary amount of time.

> The theory is that many with gut weakness find it difficult to digest multiple chain sugars.

Fruit, meats and vegetables are single chain sugars and are therefore easier on the body.

When the healing of the gut wall is complete, you can then transition to properly prepared grains and starches.

This would be soaked and sprouted grains and potatoes.

Please work closely with a trusted dietitian to provide suitable substitutes.

Ingredients

- One whole chicken, or several chicken marylands (organic is always preferred but do what you can afford).
- 1 brown onion, 2 garlic cloves, 1 celery stick, diced
- 2 carrots cut into big chunks
- One egg per bowl
- Very good squeeze of lemon
- 2 sprigs of oregano
- Pinch of salt

Making it

1. Fry onions until translucent, adding garlic, sea salt, celery and carrot into the stock-pot along with the chicken.
2. Cover with filtered water and put on a slow simmer for at least three hours.
3. Add an egg to the hot stock and stir.
4. Break apart chicken pieces and shred.
5. Serve in individual bowls and squeeze lemon into soup until it becomes cloudy

Greek-style chicken soup.

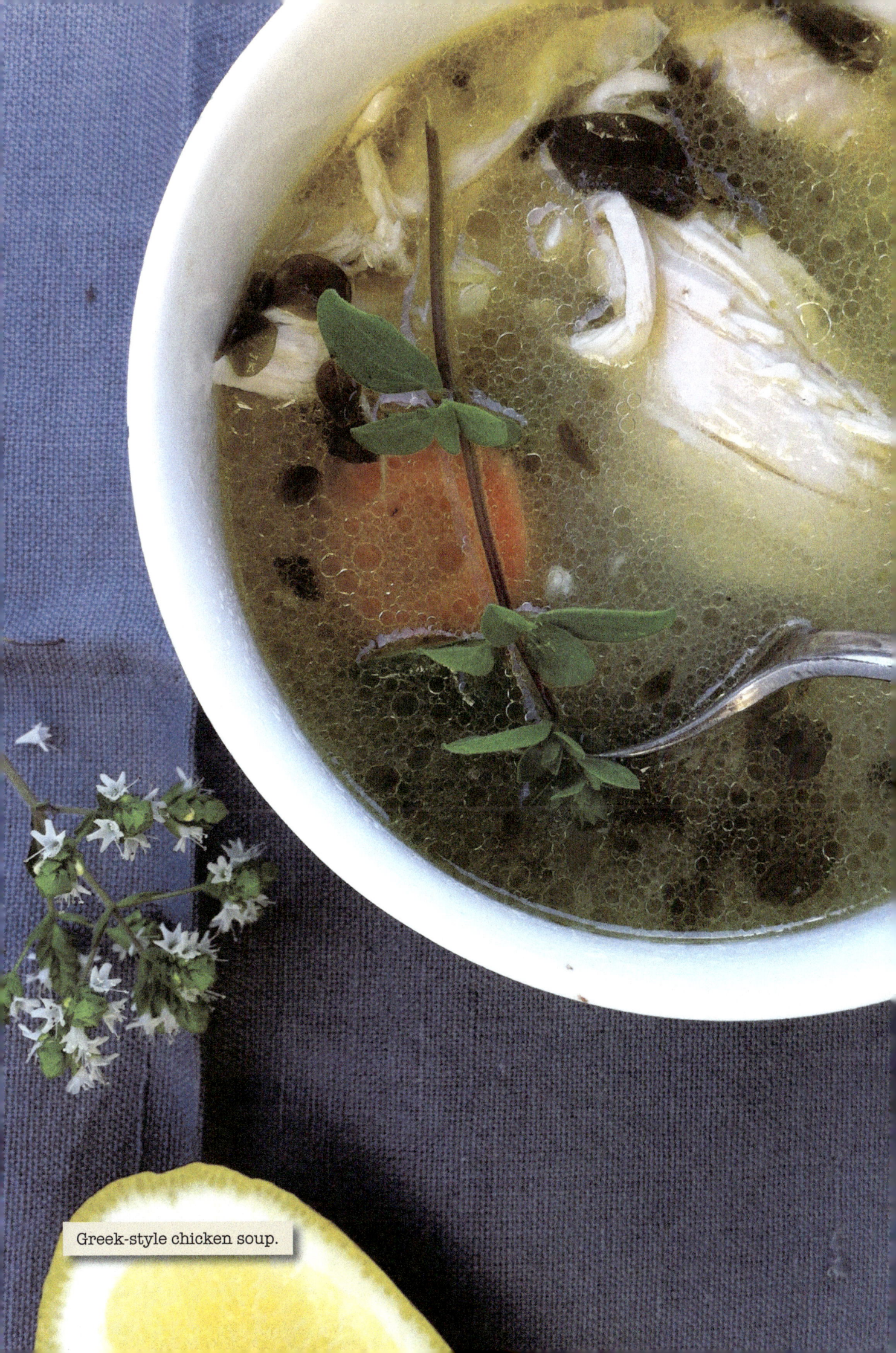

Carrot, cabbage, marjoram & chicken soup

This is the kind of thing you can make a big batch of first thing in the morning, leave it and have a meal ready in minutes at any time of the day.

Freezes well too.

For us, soup and stews are where it's at.

Healing, easy to digest and delicious.

To make it yummy I've found it's all about what you put with it.

> I always serve the soup with a drizzle of basil or garlic infused olive oil on top and a dollop of cultured cream.

Ingredients

- 1 shallot
- 1 leek
- 3 cloves garlic
- Butter, ghee or coconut oil
- Two chicken Marylands
- ¼ cabbage
- 5 carrots
- 3 sprigs marjoram
- Handful of parsley

Making it

1. Fry one finely sliced leek, shallot, and three cloves of garlic in butter or ghee until golden.
2. Add two chicken Marylands, a quarter of a cabbage finely sliced, five carrots chopped, a few sprigs of marjoram, and good handful of parsley and a pinch of salt.
3. Cover with water and bring to the boil, then let simmer for about one hour.
4. Take out chicken and de-bone. Take out sprigs or stalks of herbs.
5. Whizz with stick mixer or go rustic. Add back chicken pieces.

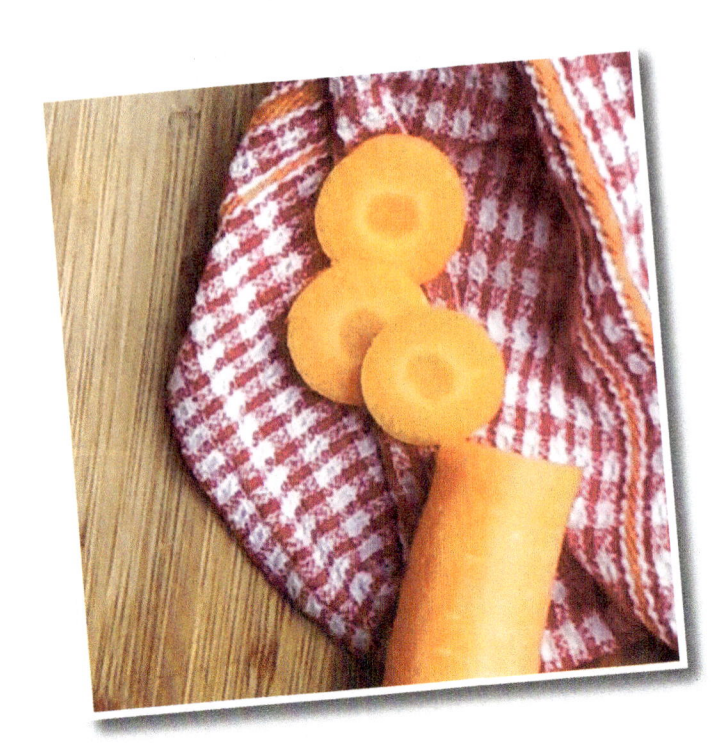

Carrot, cabbage, marjoram, chicken soup.

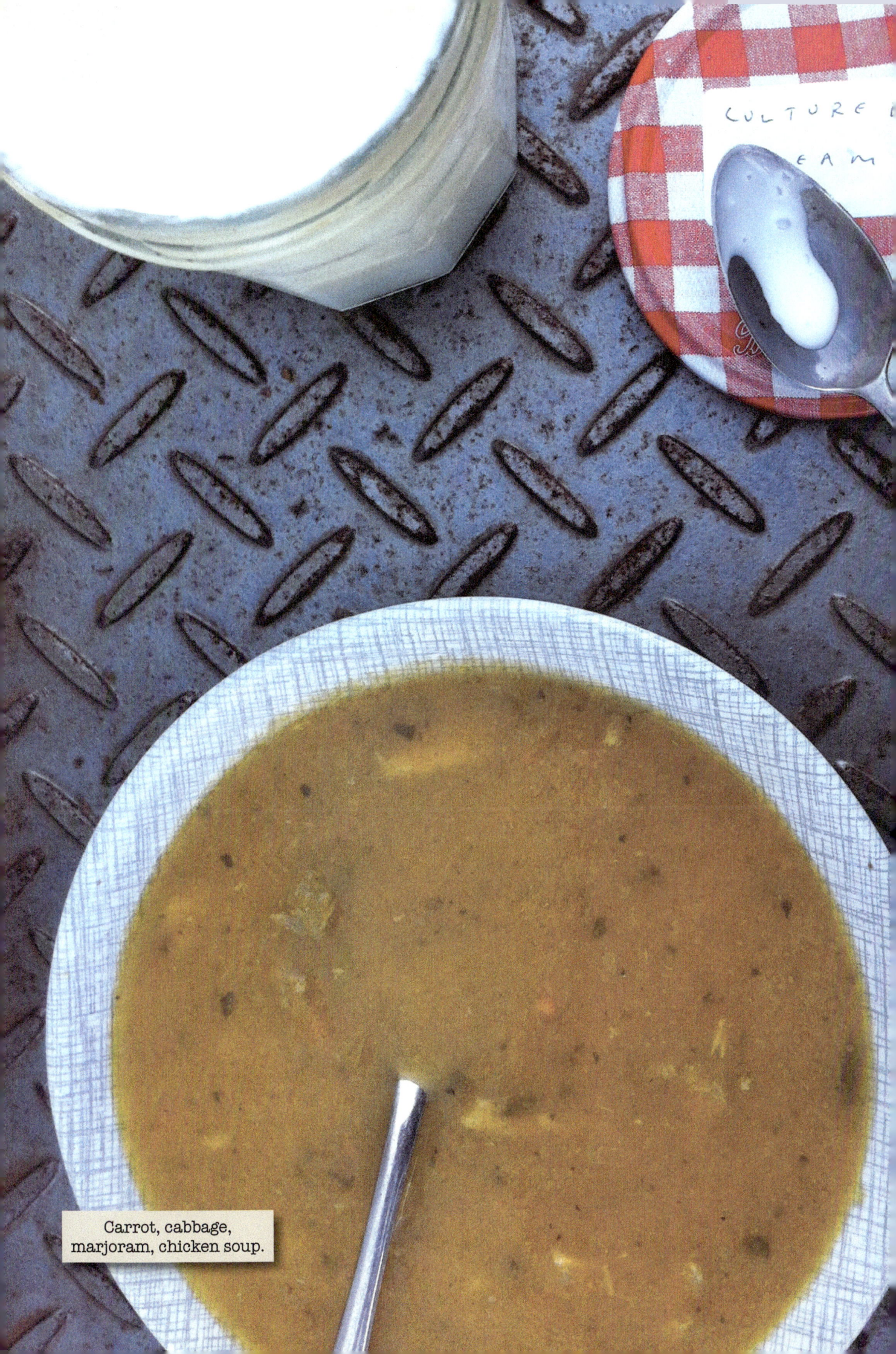

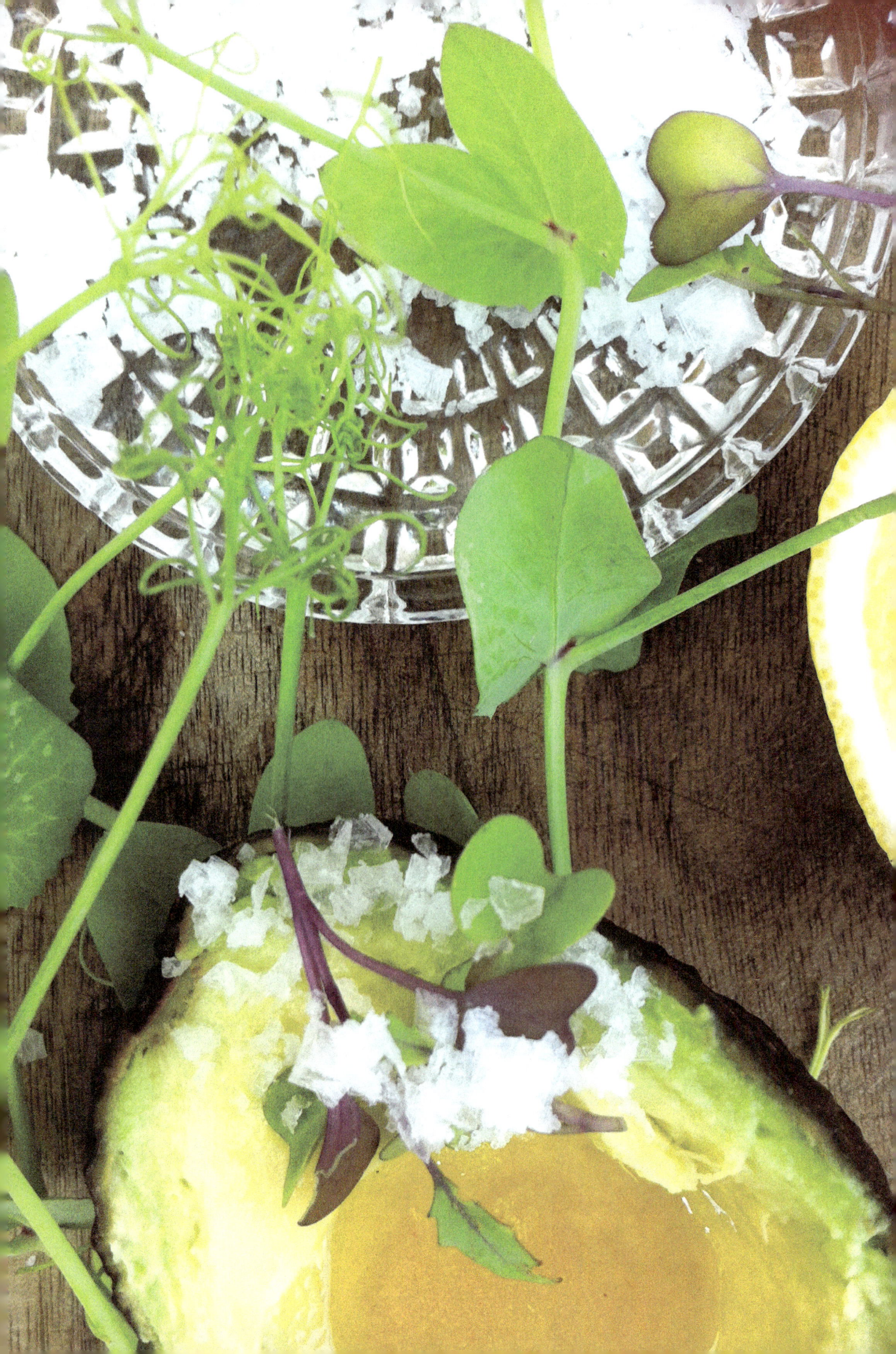

Main Meals

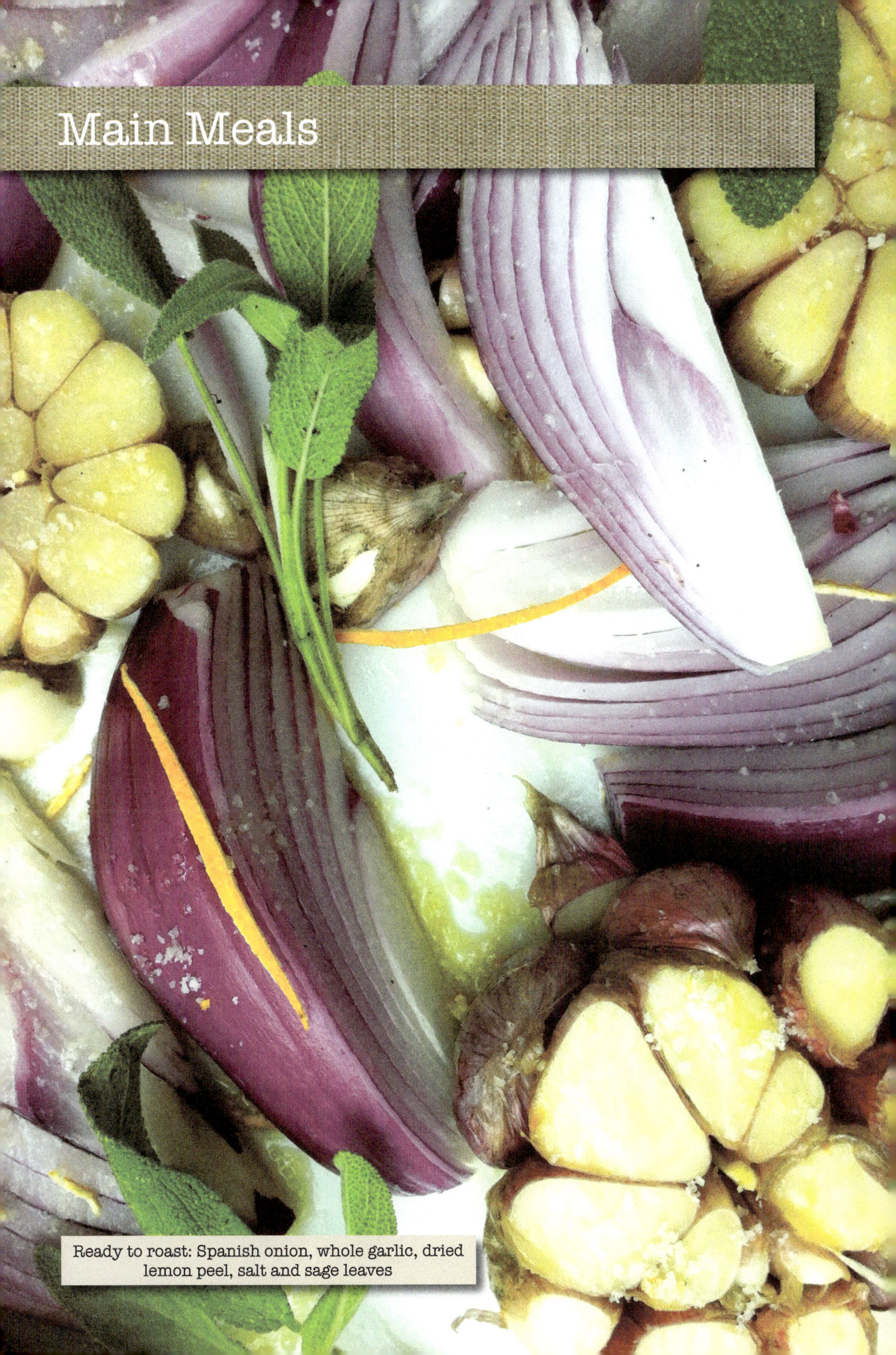

Ready to roast: Spanish onion, whole garlic, dried lemon peel, salt and sage leaves

Cauliflower mashed 'faux'tatoes, scallops & rocket micro greens.

Love potatoes. Especially mashed. But when you've got digestive weakness I have found that one of the best ways to give your belly a break is to leave out the starch for a while.

Turns out you can make all sorts of stuff out of cauli like pizza bases and wraps and if you're avoiding grains for a while it really becomes your very good friend.

Many on the autism spectrum benefit from a grain free, starch free diet.

Getting back to neurologist and nutritionist Natasha Campbell McBride. This amazing mother and doctor healed her own autistic son by being sugar, grain and starch free and believes that in many cases autism is a gut-related condition and does not have to be a permanent condition. The earlier you are able to start to heal the gut, the better the results are.

> I can only speak from my own experience, but in our case, all autistic traits that I saw in Stevie have disappeared while we are doing this diet.

They left gradually but they have gone. It has totally changed and broadened my understanding of autism. We are one example of many thousands who are experiencing the same fantastic results.

Ingredients

- 1 whole cauliflower
- Cultured cream
- Soft herbs such as basil, coriander or parsley
- Clove of garlic, chopped finely
- 12 scallops
- Micro greens (if you have them)

Making it

1. Take a whole cauliflower, break it into florets and boil in water until soft.
2. You could even boil in homemade chicken stock for an even deeper flavour.
3. Add a clove of garlic and soft herbs such as parsley, basil, spring onions.
4. Drain the cauliflower well and whizz with a stick mixer until smooth.
5. Add a generous amount of cultured cream at the end or alternatively, a knob of cultured garlic herb butter or ghee.
6. Pan-fry the freshest, plumpest scallops you can find in some ghee, butter or duck fat. This will only take a few minutes on high heat.
7. Place scallops on top of the cauliflower and season with salt and pepper, fresh olive oil and micro greens if you have them. (They are super easy to grow and packed with nutrients).

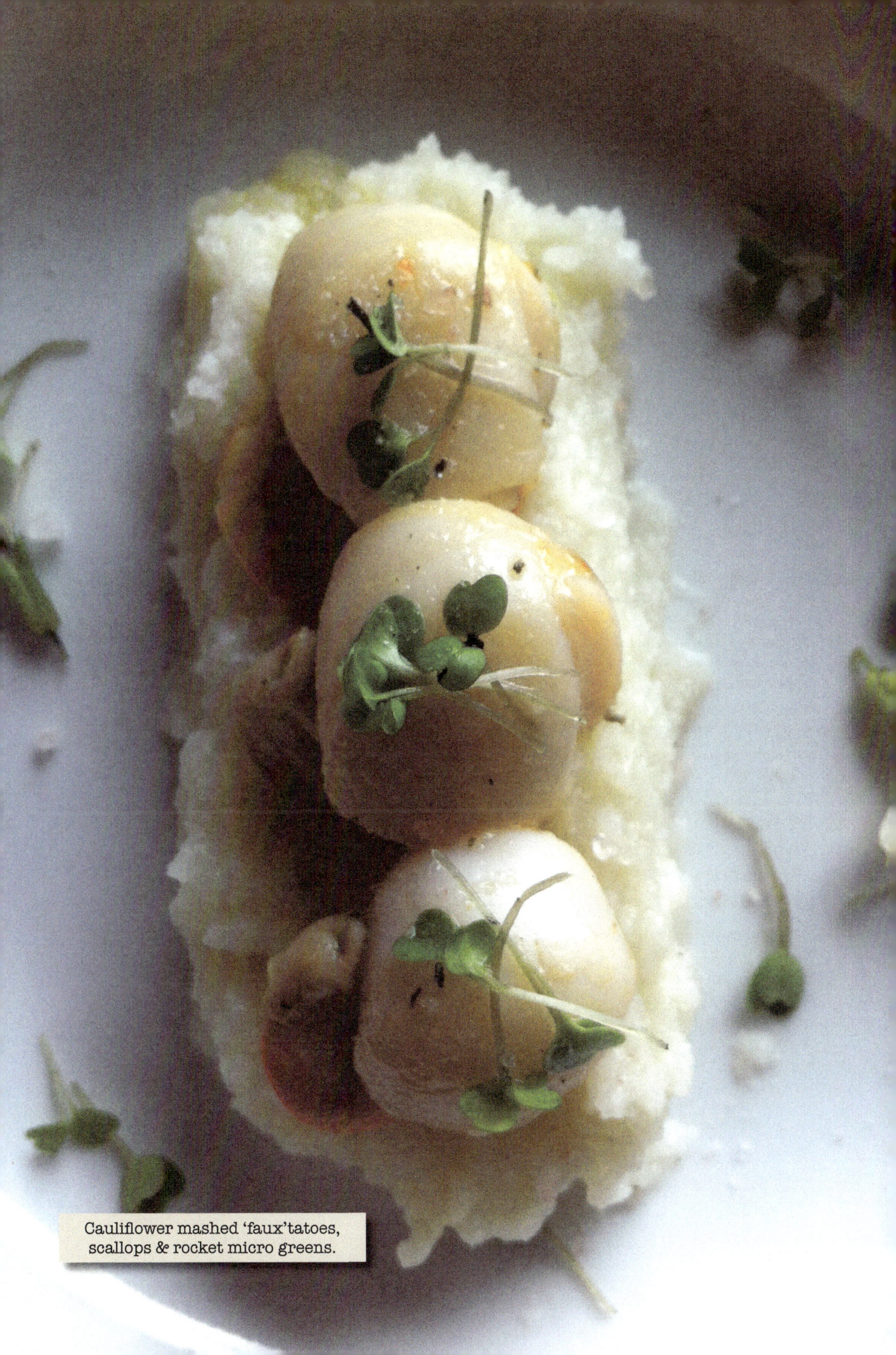

Cauliflower mashed 'faux'tatoes, scallops & rocket micro greens.

Classic Sunday roast, buttered carrots, sage & rosemary salt

With the rise of multi-culturalism in this country we are happily now pretty comfortable with a bit of dukkah on our pita and a few wantons in our soup.

But the more I learn about how digestion works, the more I realise that the traditional meat and three veg of the 50s has its wisdom.

If you are trying to make things easier on your stomach, I have found that sticking to foods that are slow cooked and ultra simple is the best thing for us.

Raw food is great if you already have a strong digestive system. It's full of enzymes and you maintain all the nutrients in a fresh, delicious form.

However, if your gut is compromised in any way, raw food can be very irritating to the gut and be very difficult to digest.

Slow cooked soups and stews and roasts can be a lot more gentle on your system.

> Think of your tummy as a pot with a fire underneath it. If you have stomach issues, often that fire is weak, rather than a big blaze.

If you then put raw, cold food into that pot, the fire has to work hard to cook it.

But if you put warm, well-cooked food into that digestive pot, there is far less work to be done.

Ingredients

- 1 whole chicken (organic wherever possible and affordable)
- ½ lemon
- 4-6 sage leaves
- 1 whole garlic bulb, 1 Spanish onion, 1 bunch whole baby carrots, 2 zucchini, ½ a pumpkin and wedges of cabbage
- 2 cups of peas to serve on the side

Making it

1. Preheat your oven to 180 degrees C.
2. Get a stainless steel or cast iron enamelled roasting pan, stuff chicken with lemon and a few garlic cloves and put it in the oven for about an hour and a half depending on the size of your chicken and the strength of your oven. Coat the sage leaves with a little ghee, butter or coconut oil and drizzle on top of the chicken.
3. About forty minutes in, add one whole garlic bulb cut in half, skin on; Spanish onion outer skin removed and cut in rustic looking chunks and all veggies apart from the peas (par boiled).
4. Drizzle the whole lot with some ghee, butter or coconut oil or duck fat if you can't do dairy and sprinkle with rosemary sea salt.
5. 20 mins in, put the peas on the stove and boil until tender and sweet.

Gravy

Ingredients

- 1 cup pan juices from roast chicken
- 2 tsp red Great Lakes Gelatine (serve hot or gravy will set)
- 1 tbs coconut flour (or sub with whizzed roasted onions)
- Squeeze of lemon
- Pinch of rosemary salt or plain salt

Making it

1. While chicken is resting collect the pan juices and put them in a small saucepan. Boil the kettle and dissolve two teaspoons of gelatine into three tablespoons of hot water, stirring quickly.
2. Add the coconut flour to pan juices and whisk quickly until smooth and well incorporated.
3. Next whisk in the gelatine and squeeze in the lemon juice. Finish with a pinch of salt.

For roast lamb, these easy condiments can go a long way towards making your meal complete.

Mint sauce

Ingredients

1 cup mint leaves

1 tsp raw honey

1 tsp apple cider vinegar

Pinch salt

Making it

1. Finely chop mint leaves.
2. Add the honey and vinegar to 1/2 cup of warm but not hot water and leave to sit for about half an hour until the flavour of the mint emerges.
3. Add more vinegar if not tart enough.

Mint jelly

Ingredients

- 1 cup mint leaves
- 1 tsp raw honey
- 1 tsp apple cider vinegar
- Pinch salt
- 2 tsp gelatine

Plan to make this in advance. It keeps well but you could make it as soon as you put your roast in and it would be good to go by the time it's ready.

Making it

1. Finely chop mint leaves.
2. Add the honey and vinegar to 1/2 cup of warm but not hot water and leave to sit for about half an hour until the flavour of the mint emerges.
3. Add more vinegar to taste if not tart enough.
4. Boil the kettle and dissolve two teaspoons of gelatine into three tablespoons of hot water, stirring quickly.
5. Add it to the mint mixture.
6. Pour into a small, glass jar and put in the fridge to set.
7. The mint may settle at the bottom of the jar but a quick stir with a teaspoon will evenly distribute it again.

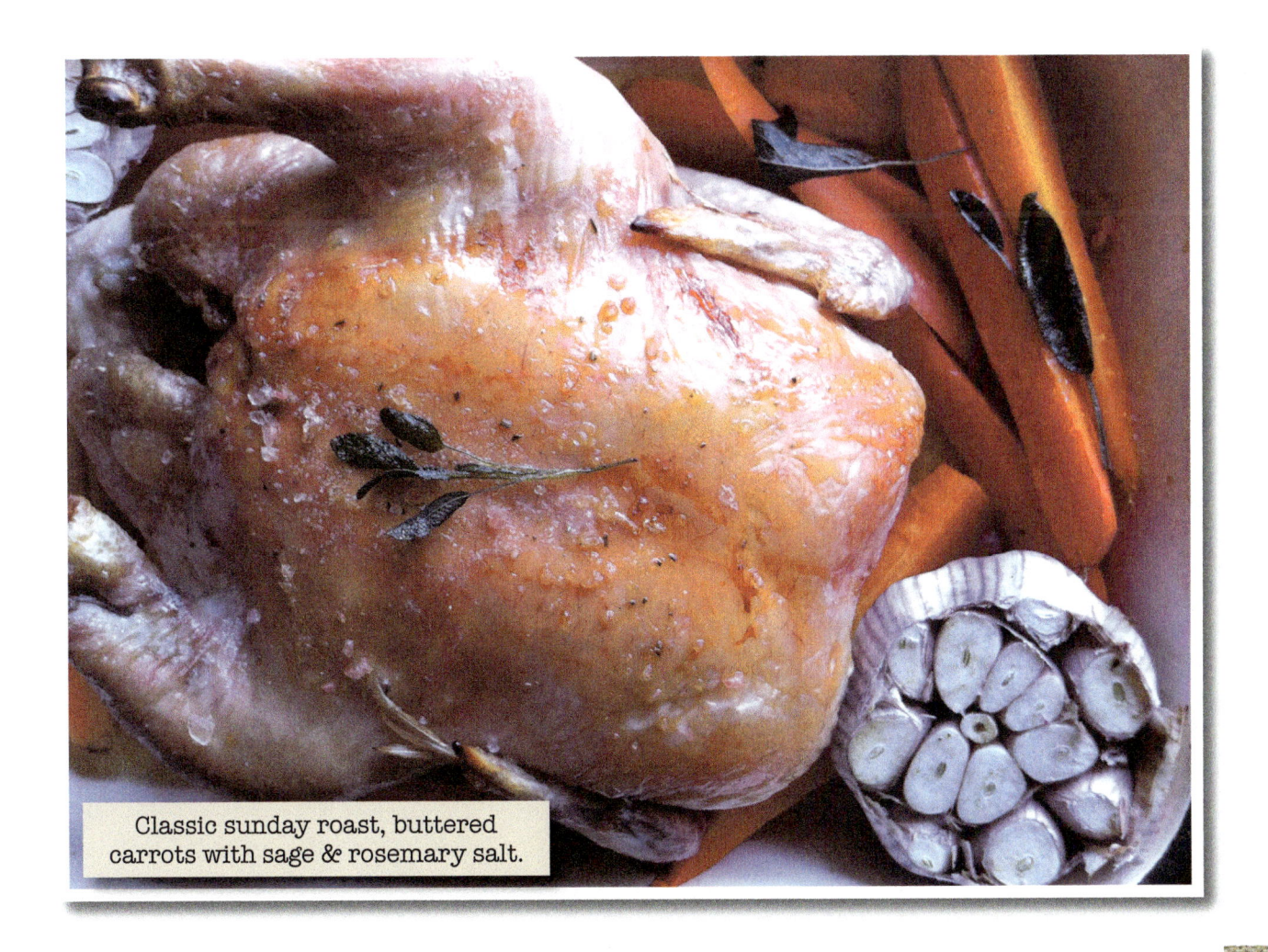

Classic sunday roast, buttered carrots with sage & rosemary salt.

French-style pickled sardines with kimchi & lime

I adapted this recipe from Rachel Khoo who you may know from the SBS series 'Little Paris Kitchen'.

The Courdon Bleu chef turned her tiny Paris apartment into one of the hottest restaurants in town. It's so tiny she can only cater for two people at a time.

Her kitchen reminds me a little of ours. It is tiny. I'm talking, one sink, tiny work bench. In fact, it came out of an old vintage caravan.

> I tell you this because I want you to know that if I can pump out meals morning, noon and night in this little kitchen, anyone can.

The tools I can't live without are my food processor, garlic press, slow cooker, stick mixer, esky, hot water bottle and juicer.

Back to Rachel now. What I love about her is her down-to-earth style and pure creativity. She's an adapter and so am I.

I also loved going back to France from my armchair here in the fishing village where I now live.

With this recipe, she uses white wine vinegar, sugar and teams her pickled sardines with a lovely cracker.

I have decided to go with apple cider vinegar and team this dish with the Korean condiment known as kimchi.

As you can see, our little 18-month-old daughter Josephine is intrigued.

Anchovies, sardines and whitebait are rich in calcium and other minerals, and vitamins A, D and B12.

They also have lower levels of mercury and other contaminants compared to larger fish.

Pan fry in butter or olive oil, coconut oil if you have a problem with dairy, strip and serve with sauerkraut or kimchi.

Ingredients

- 6 sardine fillets, de-boned (I got our fishmonger to do this for me)
- 1 cup apple cider vinegar
- 2 juniper berries (optional)
- 2 tsp raw honey
- Pinch salt
- 1 Lebanese cucumber, finely chopped
- Cultured Spanish onion, finely chopped
- Lemon and lime zest

Making it

1. Mix vinegar, raw honey (dissolved in a tbs of warm water), juniper berries and salt together and pour liquid over fish fillets in a shallow, ceramic dish until they are completely covered.
2. Cover dish completely and place in the fridge.
3. Leave this to marinate in the fridge for about 4-6 hours or overnight. Be sure to give it about an hour before serving to take the chill off.
4. When ready to serve, scatter platter with cultured onion, finely diced cucumber and lemon and lime zest.

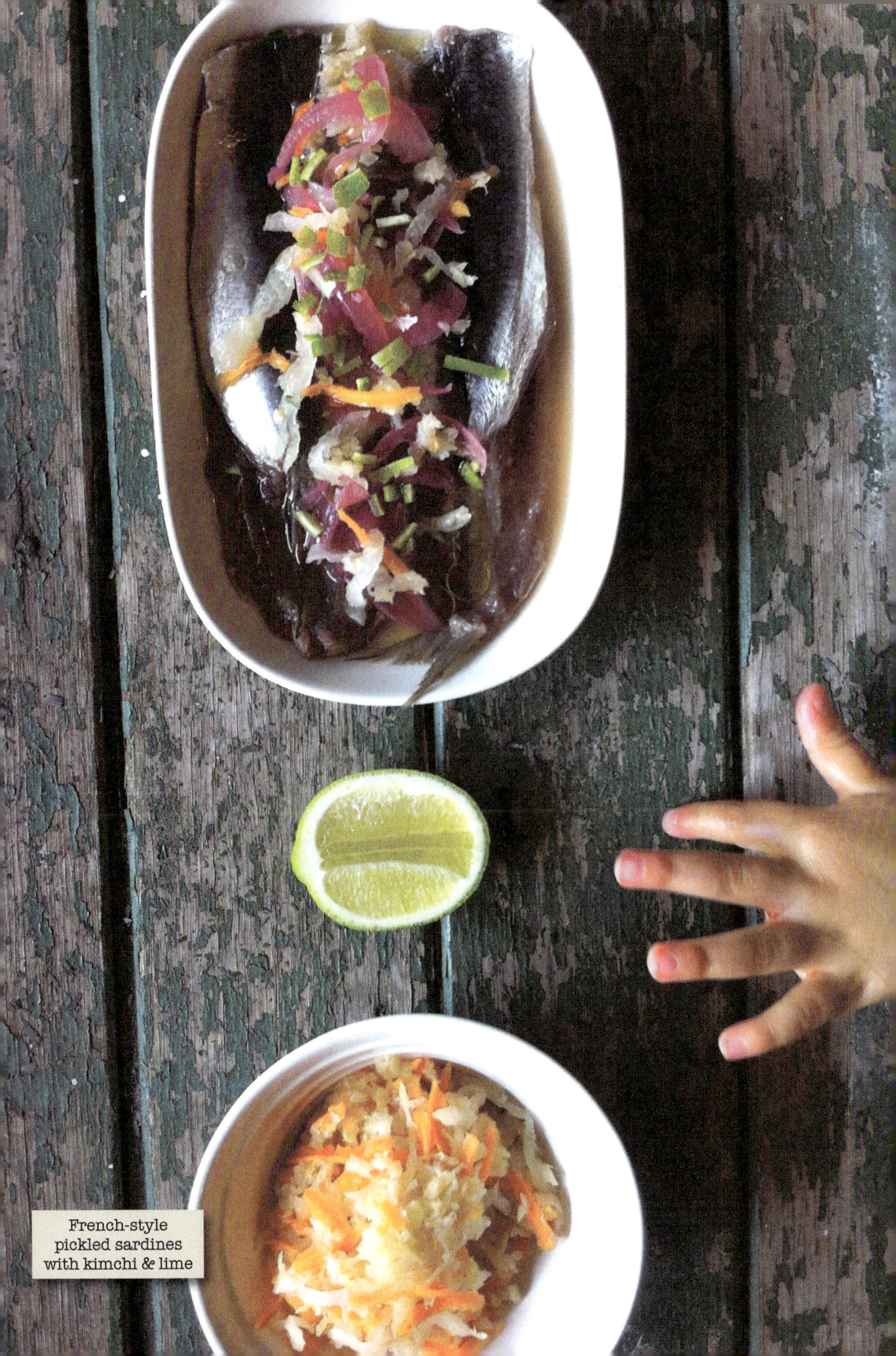

French-style pickled sardines with kimchi & lime

Sumac salted roast pork belly with sage carrots

This delicious, lemony red dust is a favourite in North Africa and loved for not only its flavour but also its medicinal properties.

Research has shown that the health benefits of sumac are many.

> Sumac works as an anti-fungal, anti-microbial, anti-oxidant and anti-inflammatory.

I like to make up a good-sized batch of sumac salt and use it on everything.

I have recently discovered that it works particularly well on roast pork belly.

Ingredients
- Pork belly
- A handful of sage leaves
- 2 tsp of Sumac salt, (see page 18)
- 1 Spanish onion or two shallots
- 1 bulb of garlic cut open sideways
- Two good handfuls of green beans, trimmed and steamed
- 1 good sized broccoli floret, broken in pieces and steamed

Making it

1. Pre-heat the oven to as high as it can go. You want the oven to be very hot to make good crackling

2. I got our butcher to score the top of the pork for us but if you are doing it yourself, get a small, very sharp knife and make scores about a cm apart into the fat. Be careful not to penetrate the meat.

3. Rub the sumac salt into all the scores.

4. Put the pork, crackling side-up, in a roasting tray big enough to hold a whole lot of vegetables and place in the hot oven for about 15-30 minutes or until the skin of the pork has started to crackle and brown. Check every 10 minutes or so. Our old fashioned oven needed about 30 minutes.

5. Turn the heat down to 180 C, add the par boiled carrots and any other vegetables you fancy.

    Spanish onions or shallots and open cut bulbs of garlic are some of my favourites and look so pretty when serving.

6. Top with seven or eight sage leaves and roast for another 1.5 hours. Cooking time varies depending on weight and size of the cut. A good butcher will be able to advise.

When done, the crackling should be golden brown and pork well cooked inside.

7. Serve with some home made mustard (page 16) and greens such as broccoli and green beans.

8. You could also make a lovely gravy for this dish using the pan juices and a sprinkle of coconut flour to thicken.

Use this kind of flour sparingly as it is very dense.

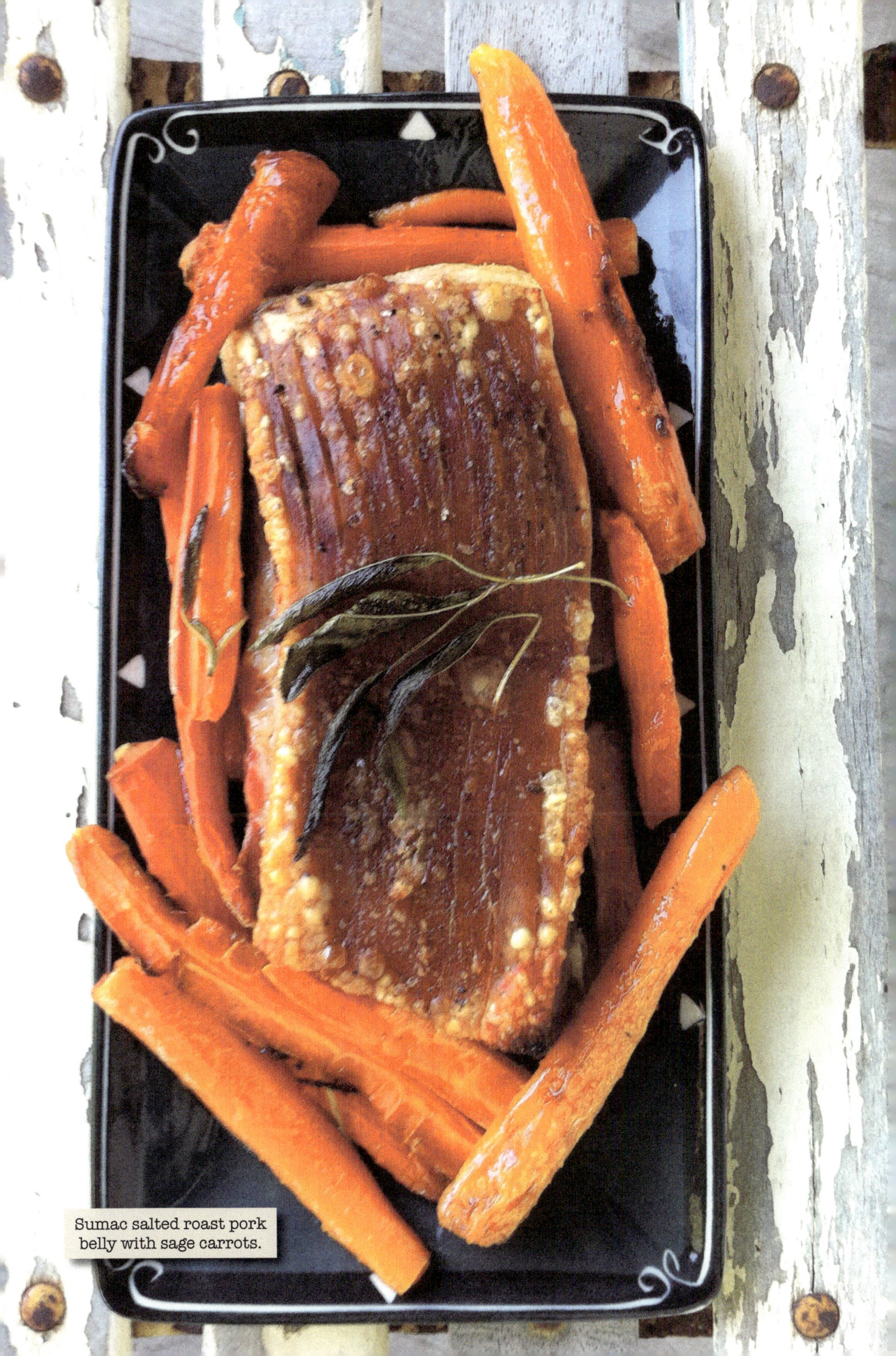

Sumac salted roast pork belly with sage carrots.

Fish with radish & fennel

As for this recipe, I put it together on one of those stinking hot days over Christmas in Australia. I wanted very minimal stove time.

I find flat head and snapper good, clean options. They cook in about three minutes in a fry pan, my kids like their mild flavour and I like them because they are not farmed, fed pellets, high in mercury etc.

We all loved this salad. I hope you do too.

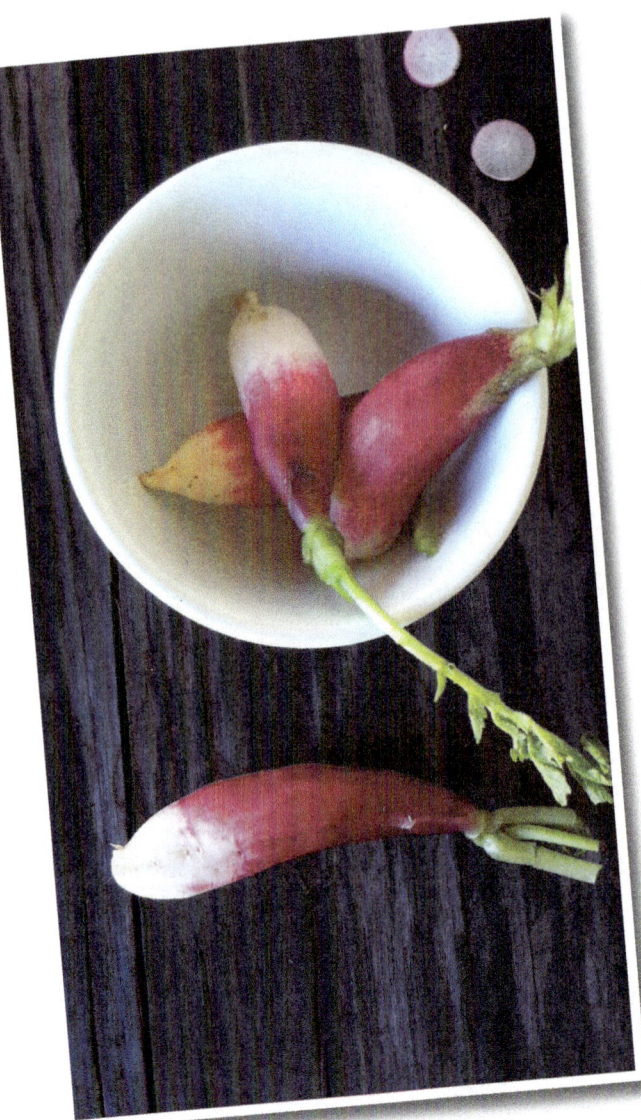

Ingredients

- Four large fish fillets
- 1 bulb fennel
- 2 radishes
- ¼ cup cultured red onion (use uncultured if you don't have it)
- 1 avocado
- 2 cups mixed lettuce leaves (very easy to grow in pots in your garden)

Making it

1. To make this, I just pan-fried the fish in a little butter or ghee.
2. With a potato peeler, I shaved fennel, radish and red onion.
3. Add avocado, lettuce if you wish, cultured vegetables like a sauerkraut give it a lovely kick - as well as the added bonus of powerful probiotics.
4. I topped this salad with some fennel tops taken from my Dad's garden. I am discovering that many vegetable leaves are full of flavour and nutrition.
5. Squeeze lemon liberally over salad.
6. Finish with the best olive oil you can find. Most olive oil you buy from supermarkets is old and has lost their flavour. It stands to reason that there are also more nutrients in fresh produce too.

Pan fried snapper salad with radish and fennel.

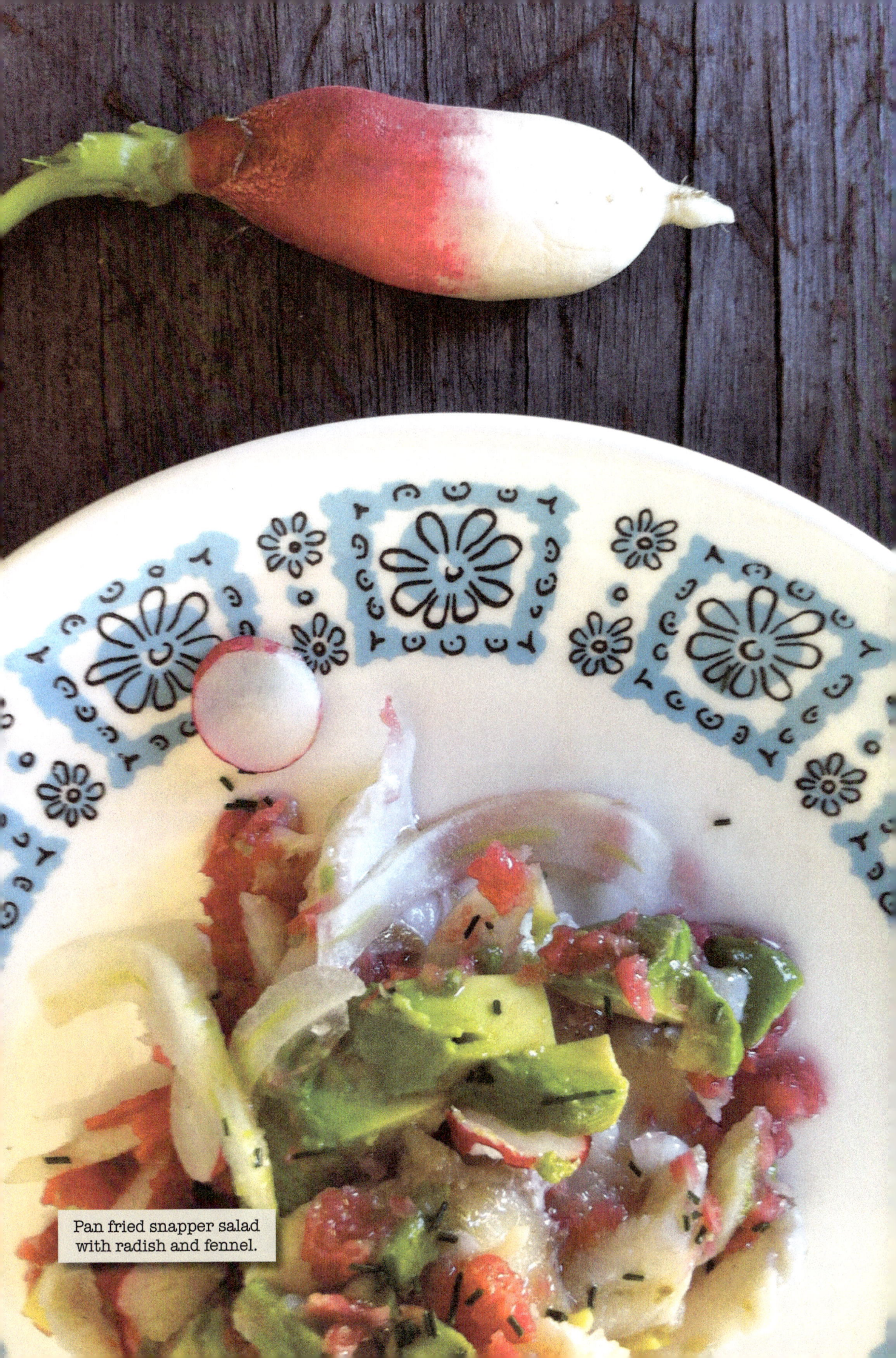

Honeyed roast chicken with tarragon, turnips, garlic & peas

This time I wanted to see if roasting the turnip and sweetening with honey would appeal to my children.

Sadly, it did not.

There is still a slight bitterness to the turnip that is a big ask of little ones. I haven't given up though. I really liked the flavour, so perhaps it's a more grown ups dish for now.

The positive news is that I tried this dish again with roasted swedes. This went down a treat with the whole family. I even got a muffin tray and finely peeled, buttered slices of swede and layered them in the pan. The result, gorgeous, crunchy little swede stacks. Roast them alongside your chicken for about an hour or until golden.

Ingredients

- 4 chicken Marylands
- 4 swedes, turnips, beets, carrots or peas
- 6 cloves of garlic
- 1 tbs of raw honey (less is fine)
- 1 tablespoon of chopped tarragon (use any soft herb if you don't have tarragon. Parsley is a great one).

Making it

1. To do this dish I put a few chicken Marylands in a roasting dish and got them started in the oven.
2. I then peel, cut turnips or swedes into wedges and par boiled them with a pinch of salt.
3. Add them to the chicken, along with some garlic cloves still in their skins and drizzle with a combination of a tbs of honey, butter or ghee and salt.
4. Scatter the whole lot with tarragon.
5. Bake in the oven at about 180 degrees for about an hour - or until golden brown.

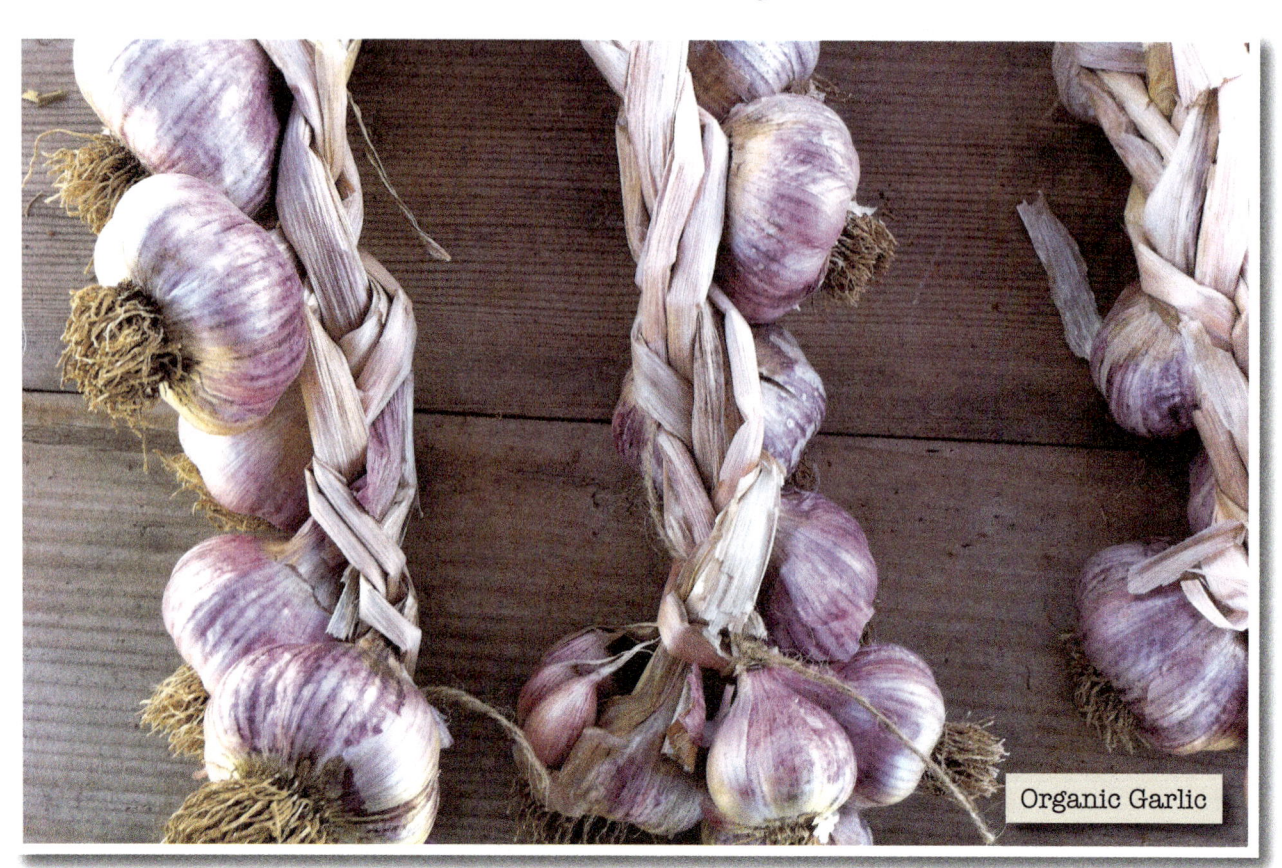

Organic Garlic

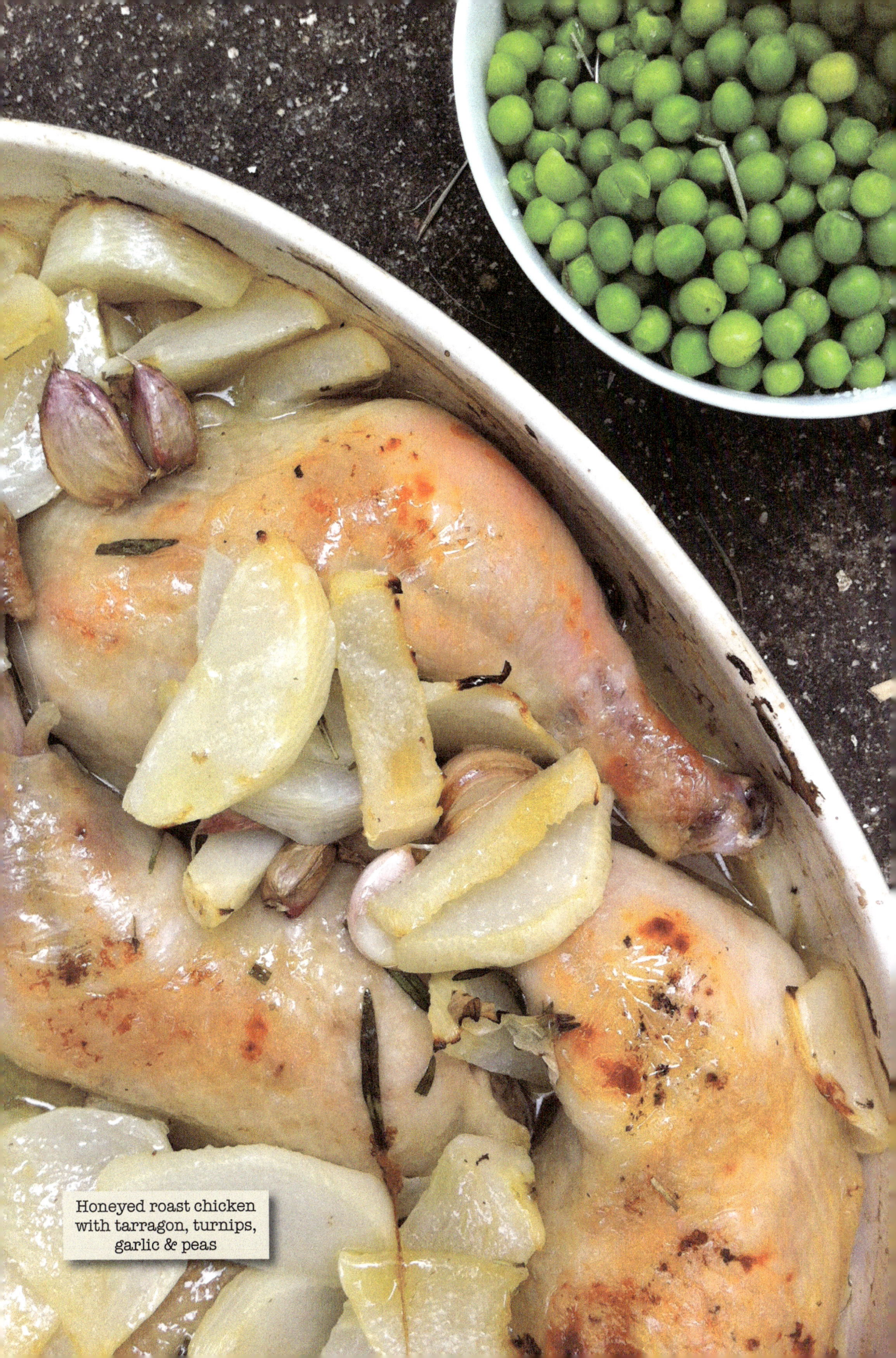

Honeyed roast chicken with tarragon, turnips, garlic & peas

Roasted swede stacks

These little roast swede stacks make for a very warming and comforting side to pork belly or roast lamb.

Swedes become sweet when slow roasted and are very popular in our house.

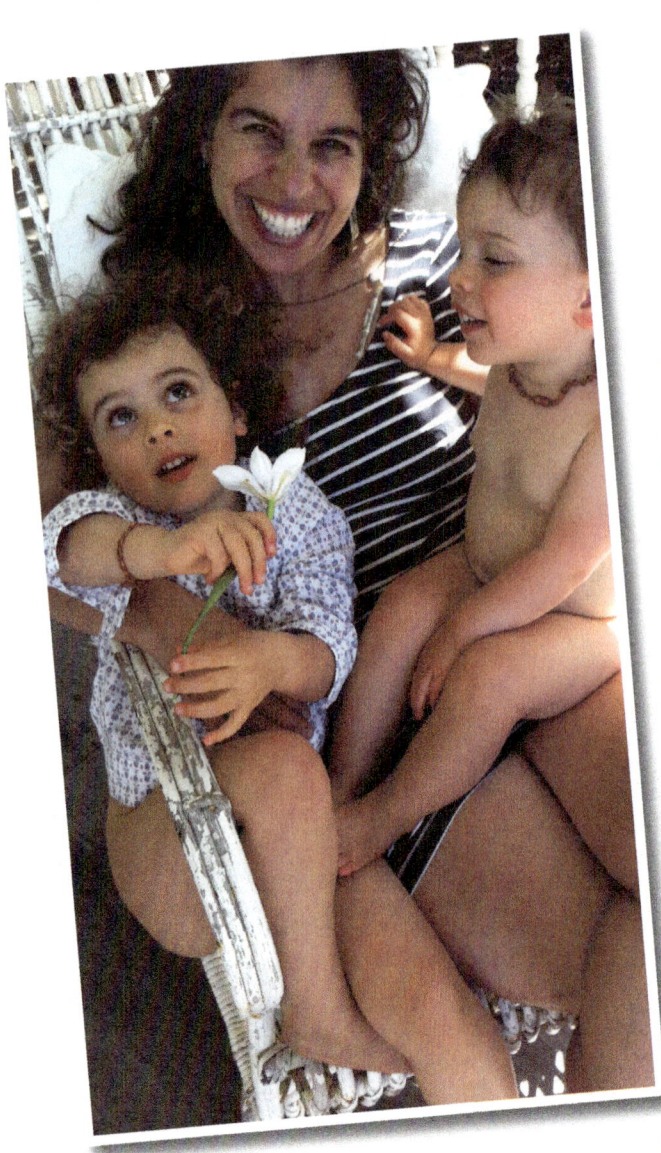

Ingredients

- 3 medium sized swedes
- Sprinkle of salt
- Butter, duck fat or lard or tallow if needing a dairy free option

Making them

1. Par boil and slice the swedes into rounds using a knife or mandolin.
2. Grease a muffin pan (use butter, duck fat or lard or tallow if needing a dairy free option).
3. Sprinkle with salt, add a few more dollops of butter on top and bake at 180 degree C for 25 mins.
4. Take out and flip the stack so that the underside becomes the top and gives the top a chance to become golden brown.
5. Serve piping hot.

Extra tips

Bulk Cooking to get you out of the kitchen and back to your family

Set aside a block of time for your cooking

Personally, I like to set aside an hour or two on a Sunday around 4pm. It's when I can get James to help out in the kitchen while the girls watch a movie or he takes the girls out to the beach or park while I can do some cooking uninterrupted. Win/win.

Variety is the spice of life

It's not just about making bigger quantities of a dish but also about using your kitchen time and space to make a variety of meals and snacks for the week. That means oven going, hob, slow cooker, things setting in the fridge and ferments on the bench top.

An hour of power

If I can't face a big cook up on the weekend, the other option I like is to set aside an hour first thing in the morning a day and do a batch of cooking for the entire day. Breakfast, lunch, dinner, snacks and drinks all happen in that hour of power. That could mean banana pancakes for brekky, chook soup for lunch, a watermelon jelly for snacks and lamb cass with cauli mash for dinner. It also means the majority of the washing up is all done and the only thing left to do is heat up and serve.

Roasted swede stacks.

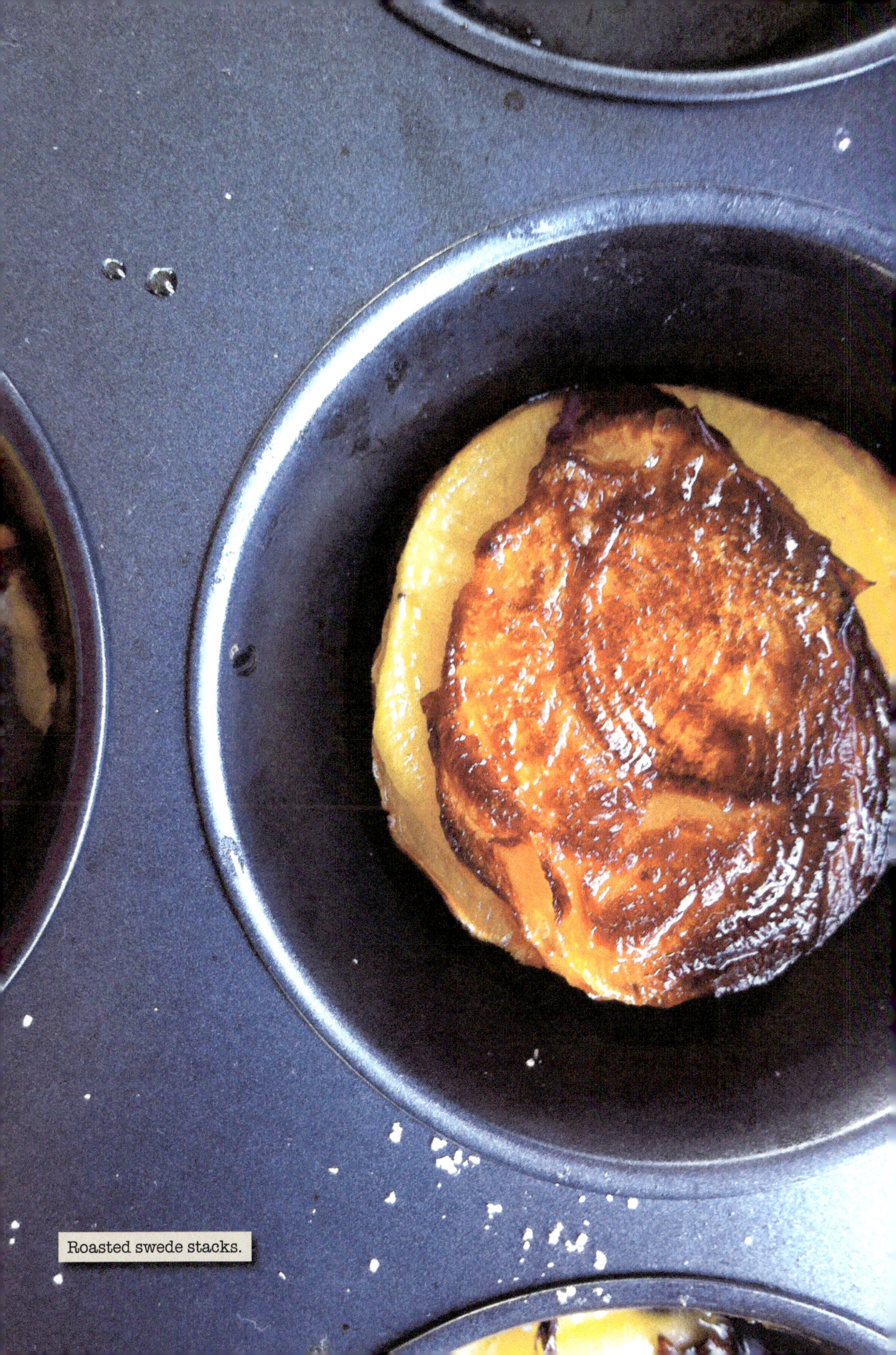

Chicken casserole with herb 'pesto'

This is a great way to get members of the onion family into your diet.

The onion is a great healer and immune system booster.

I don't do quantities most of the time when cooking. One of my mum's greatest gifts is to have taught me to cook by feel. It has made it easier for me in the long run.

It's about getting a sense of what flavours go together.

Today, this casserole is full of leek, garlic, shallots and finished with what I call pesto.

Although it does not include any parmesan or pine nuts, I chop about a cup of herbs finely, add garlic pressed through a press, and then add olive oil.

Depending on where you are at with your gut health, add activated sunflower seeds or nuts to this mix, finely chopped (I use a mezza luna). I've also added a few dates well chopped in the past and it is amazing. For those doing the GAPS Diet, please omit the dates.

> Right now we are having fruit on its own rather than with the main meal because it makes the digestive system work harder but those who are further along with their healing will love it.

I put this pesto on top of most of our food and my kids eat it without question, whereas if the garlic was a little thicker they would reject it and its hot, pungent quality.

Raw garlic is a great natural anti-parasitic. Have a garlic-heavy pesto like this when you are sick with a cold. It knocks our colds right out of our systems.

Ingredients

- 4 chicken Marylands
- 1 leek or two shallots finely chopped
- 2 garlic cloves, pressed
- 1 tbs butter, ghee, coconut oil for frying
- 2 cups diced pumpkin
- 1 cup peas
- 1 zucchini
- 3 carrots
- 1 tsp salt
- 1 tbs soft herbs
- Water or home made stock to cover ingredients

Making it

1. For this cass, I chop leek, garlic, shallot finely and fried in butter, ghee or any other animal fat (duck fat would be yum) until soft.
2. I then add diced pumpkin and frozen organic peas, a zucchini and three carrots.
3. Cover it all with chicken stock (home made only) and whatever herbs I have in the garden (this time I used spring onion and chives).
4. I threw in about a tsp of salt (Himalayan pink salt is so delicious).
5. I then had some chicken that I had cooked in our slow cooker so I put that in and put the lid on. Simmer for about 30 mins and let most of the liquid reduce.
6. If you are starting with uncooked chicken, just brown it in the pot after your leeks and shallots. Depending on the cut of meat it will take more time. Bone in meat, give it a good hour.
7. Serve with home made yoghurt and pesto on top.

Chicken casserole with herb 'pesto'

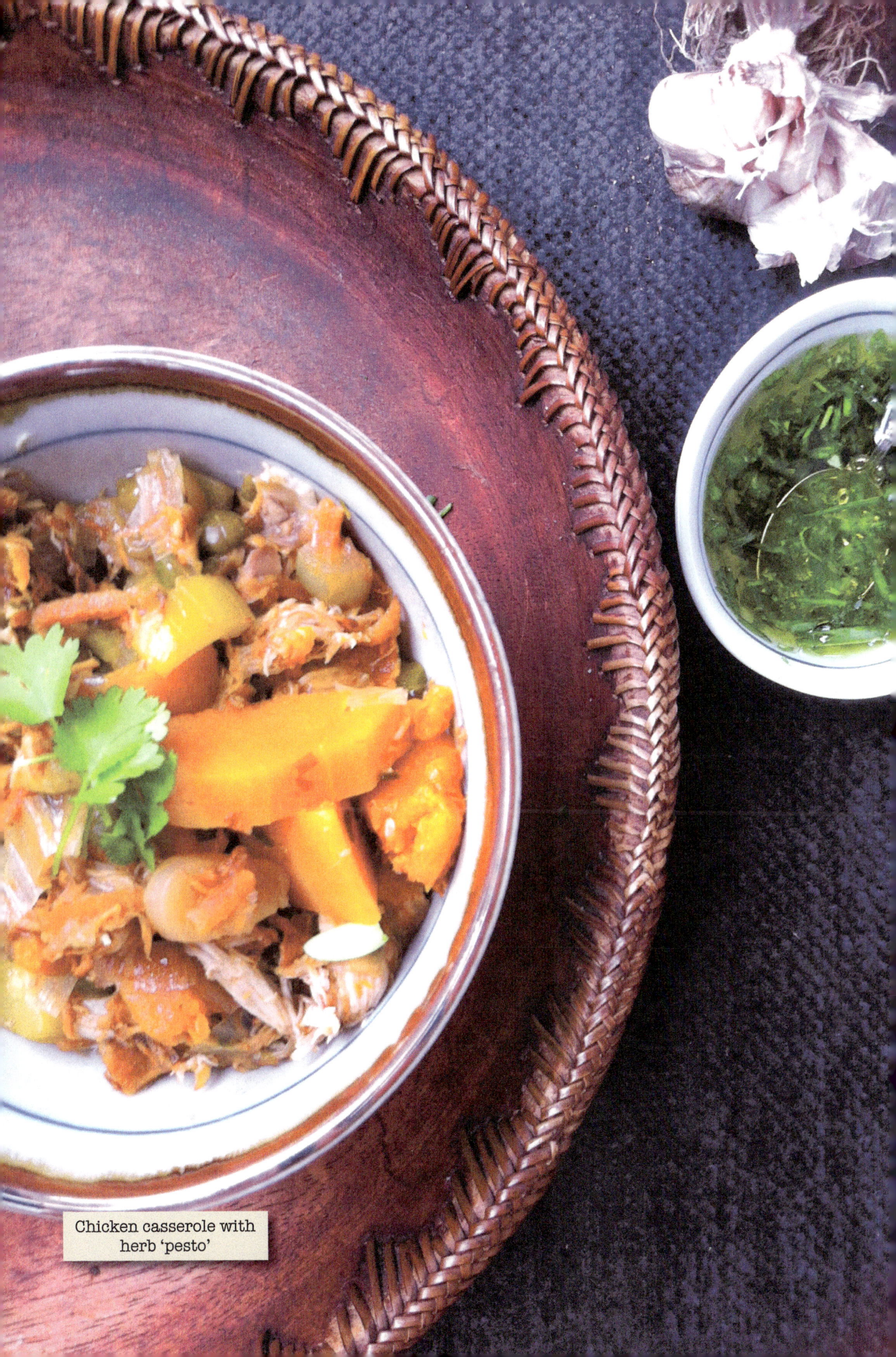

Greek style lamb cutlets, home made yoghurt with mint, sauerkraut & pumpkin chips

Why? Because on a hot day I want something my kids love that I can put together in about three minutes.

Also because lamb is rich in zinc, yoghurt - a natural probiotic and sauerkraut - a very powerful probiotic too.

Always sauerkraut in our house. Packed with enzymes, this incredible food, which dates back to Genghis Khan, helps to digest meats and fats.

Start with a teaspoon and work up. It's powerful stuff. According to Wikipedia:

"Fermented foods have a long history in many cultures. Today, two of the most well-known instances of traditional fermented cabbage side dishes are sauerkraut and Korean kimchi.

The Roman writers Cato (in his De Agri Cultura), and Columella (in his De re Rustica), mentioned preserving cabbages and turnips with salt.

It is believed to have been introduced to Europe in its present form 1,000 years later by Genghis Khan after invading China.

The Tartars took it in their saddlebags to Europe. There it took root mostly in Eastern European and Germanic cuisines, but also in other countries including France, where the name became choucroute.

Before frozen foods, refrigeration, and cheap transport from warmer areas became readily available in northern and central Europe, sauerkraut, like other preserved foods, provided a source of nutrients during the winter.

James Cook always took a store of sauerkraut on his sea voyages, since experience had taught him it prevented scurvy."

Ingredients

- 8 lamb cutlets or mid loin chops (can be pricey so any lamb cuts suitable for frying are fine)
- 1 tbs chopped oregano
- ½ lemon
- ½ butternut pumpkin
- 1 cup yoghurt
- 2 tbs mint
- 1 clove raw garlic (optional)

Making it

1. Fry lamb covered in chopped oregano in a frypan with a tsp of butter, ghee or coconut oil until brown and just pink in the middle.
2. Allow to rest while making the pumpkin chips.
3. When ready to serve, finish with a squeeze of lemon juice.

Pumpkin chips

1. Slice a butternut pumpkin finely.
2. Fry with butter/ghee/ duck fat or coconut oil until golden. Or if not a hot day, make an hour ahead by baking in the oven.
3. Season with Herbs de Provence salt, or any salt you have on hand.

Yoghurt mint dip

1. I was making a small quantity so for this I took a mezza luna (a half moon knife and board with a hole in it) and chopped a handful of the mint finely.
2. I then poured a cup of homemade yoghurt into a bowl and pressed one clove of raw garlic through a garlic press.
3. Mix it all together, add a squeeze of lemon, a pinch of salt and a slug of olive oil to finish.

Sauerkraut

I always try to serve meals with a cultured veggie.

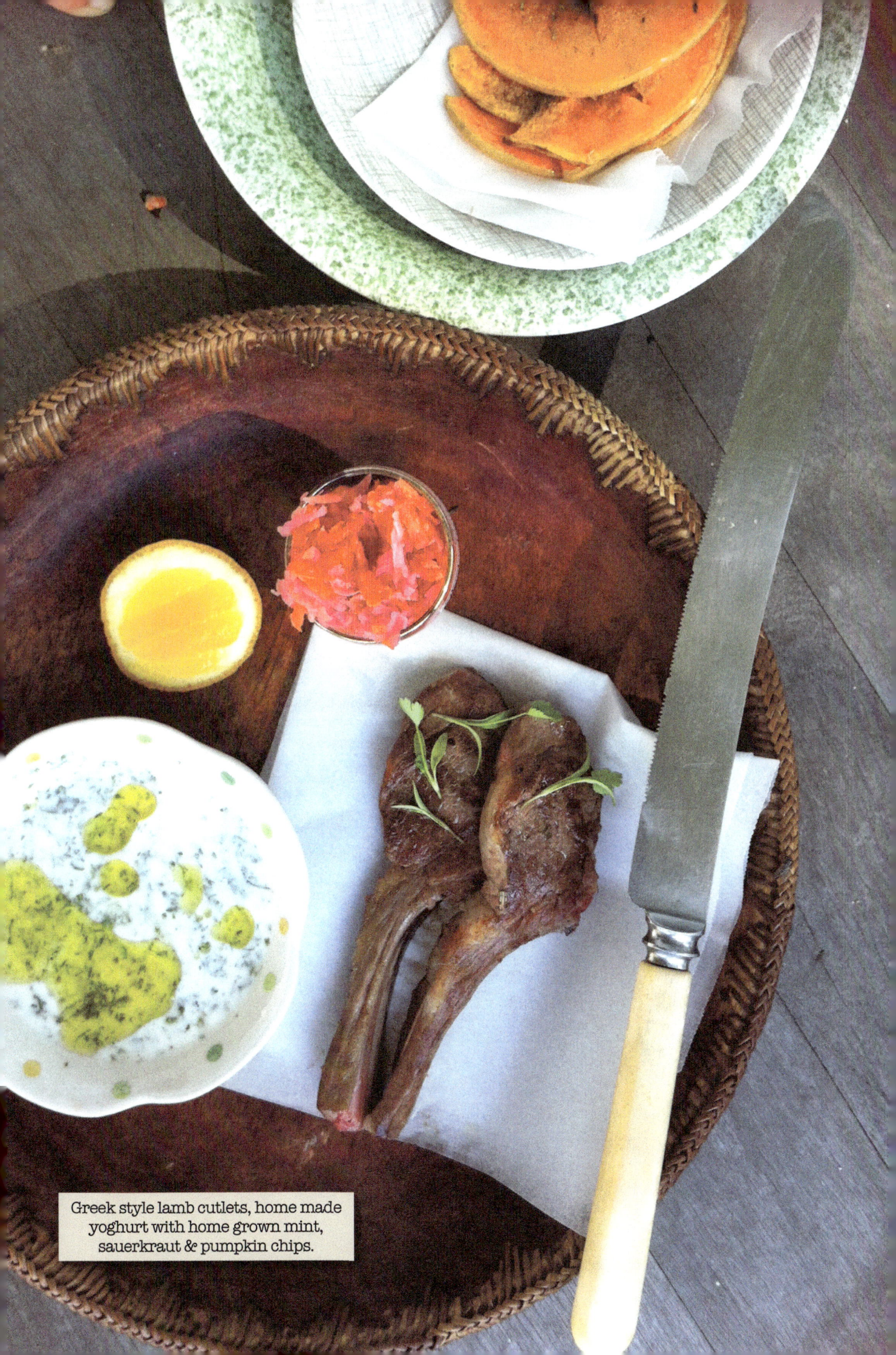

Greek style lamb cutlets, home made yoghurt with home grown mint, sauerkraut & pumpkin chips.

That classic combination – fish & chips by the beach.

We never regret an early evening run on the beach. It gives us a reset, and reminds us all how lucky we are.

As I see my children running on the beach, healthy, vital, I feel total happiness.

Everyone is famished after some time on the sand.

Fish is super quick. I have big jars of cultured veggies to make my salads. On this day, all there was to do was experiment with turnip chips. We are avoiding potatoes for now.

Their starchy quality, as beautiful and comforting as it is can be hard to digest.

We wanted something crunchy to go with some lovely flat head tails we got from our local fishmonger.

I peeled the turnip and cut into shoestrings with a mandolin. I fried with coconut oil. For those doing the GAPS Diet, frying with olive oil is not recommended, as it doesn't cope with such high temperatures.

Ghee would also work beautifully here. Handles the high temps no sweat. Drain on paper towel and sprinkle with rosemary salt.

I patted dry our fish fillets with paper towel and then coated them in a mix of coconut flour, salt, and chives. Some people report good success by whisking in an egg to this mixture.

Again, fry quickly on both sides until cooked through.

Serve with tri-coloured cultured salad and drizzle with the best, freshest olive oil you can buy - don't skimp on this. Remember, food is medicine.

Verdict: Kids liked and then did not like. I liked very much.

I have since done the same with swede chips with a much more positive reception. Swede chips it is then.

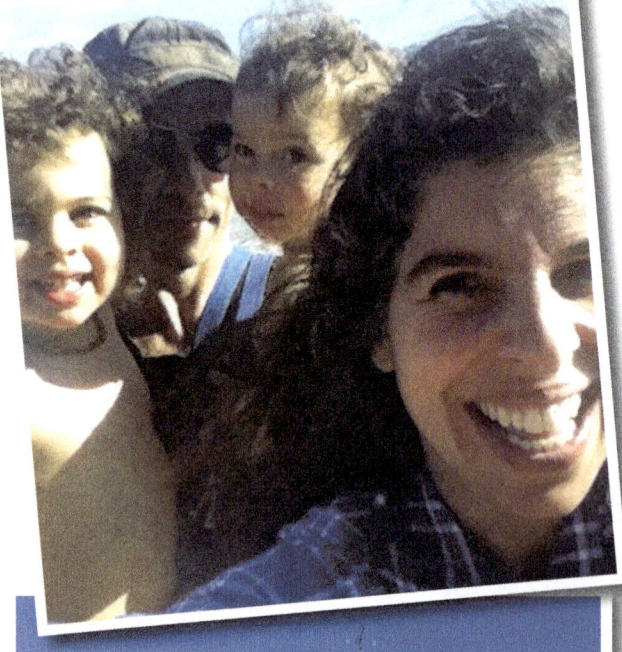

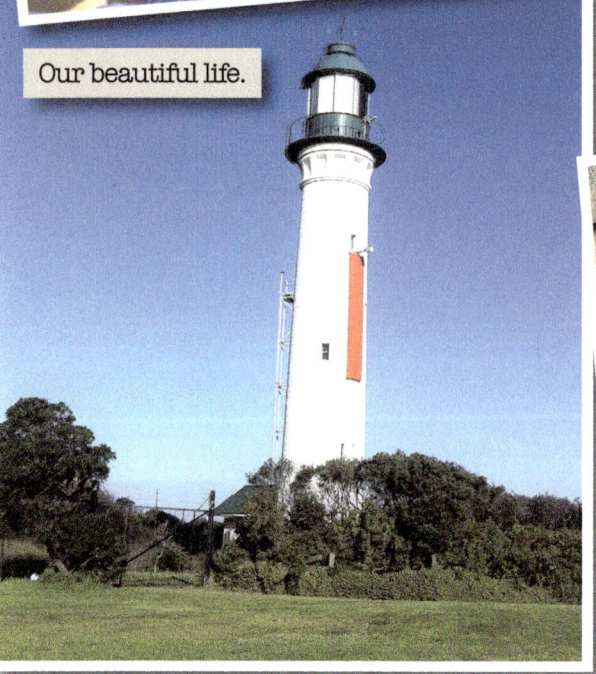

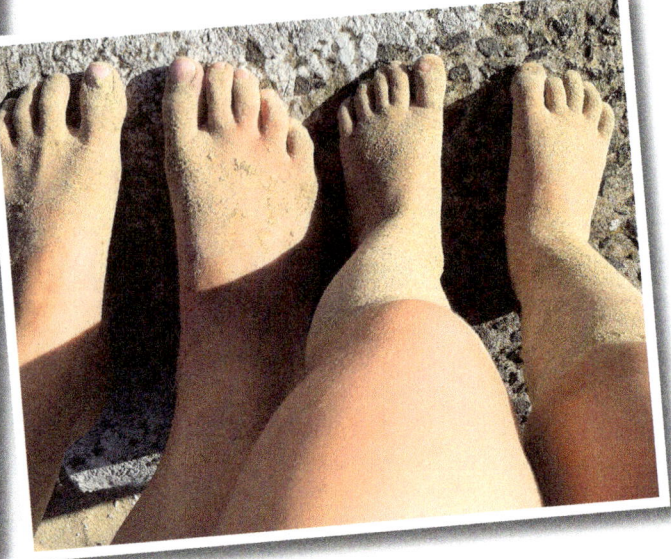

Our beautiful life.

Fish & chips.

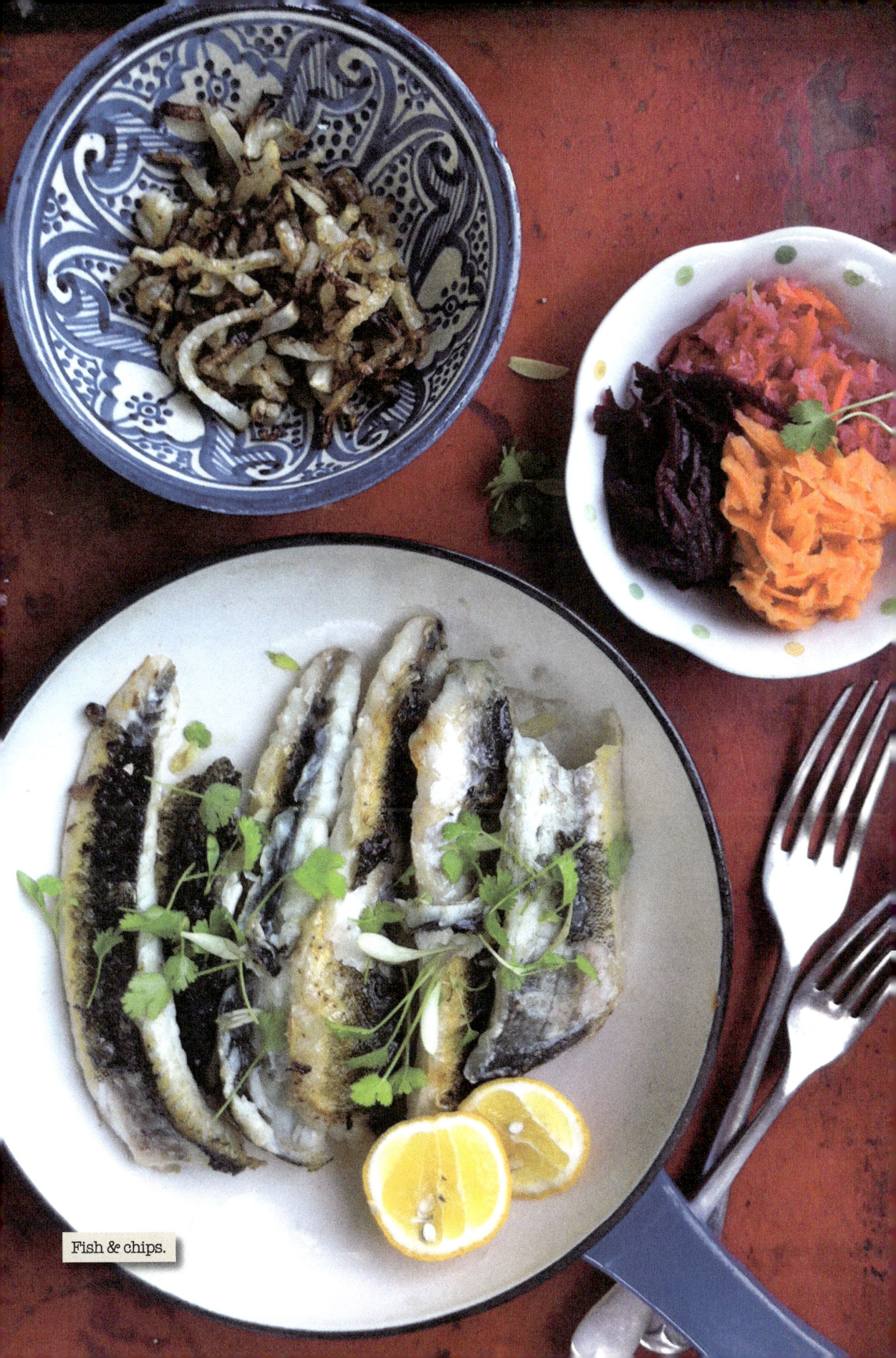

Scallops, cultured cream & herbs

These are a super quick lunchtime fix.

Scallops are not only delicious but they are high in zinc.

Many people with digestive complaints tend to be low in this essential mineral, which can affect their sleep and ability to tolerate certain foods among other things.

Serve with roquette leaves (easy and quick to grow in a pot), olive oil and sauerkraut.

Ingredients

- 6 scallops per person
- 1 tsp of ghee for frying
- 2 tbs of freshly chopped herbs, basil, parsley, spring onions – whatever you can grow in your garden.

Making it

1. In a hot fry pan with ghee, add very fresh scallops and allow to sear on each side for only a few minutes each.
2. Place fry pan in the middle of the table or serve individually with freshly chopped herbs, basil, parsley, spring onions – whatever you can grow in your garden.

Extra tip

If you do nothing else, grow a kitchen herb garden. Do not underestimate the healing power and flavour of these wonderful plants.

Even if you have no garden and no balcony at all, you can still grow micro herbs on your windowsill.

Basil and coriander work especially well - full of youthful flavour and packed with nutrients.

You can also try sprouting your own broccoli seeds for a burst of super high nutrition.

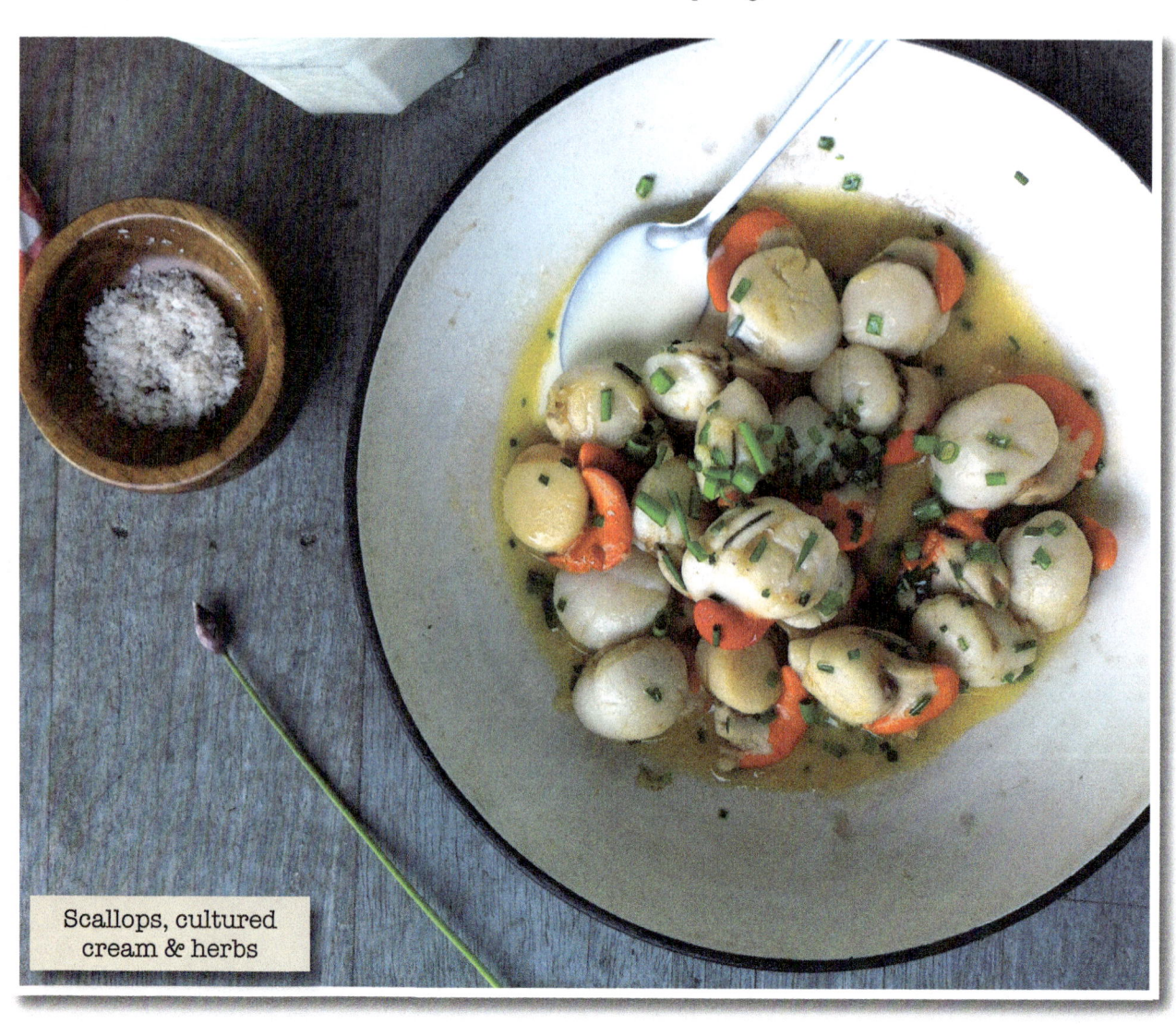

Scallops, cultured cream & herbs

Sweets for My Sweet

Raspberry tarts in the making.

Apple, orange, macadamia & date crumble

This is the only dessert I can make with my eyes closed.

I make it when our children go to bed and I have a craving for something sweet but don't have any energy left. I eat this sugar free treat again when I wake up in the morning.

It is easily subbed to make a nut free dessert by omitting the macadamia and using sunflower seeds which you can grind into a flour in a coffee grinder very quickly and easily.

> Incidentally, I have finally discovered zest. A little goes a long way and it is amazing in this kind of dish.

For those doing the GAPS Diet, desiccated coconut is something for after the introductory phase of the protocol.

I have experimented leaving it out to make it suitable for those on the introduction phases of the diet and it works beautifully.

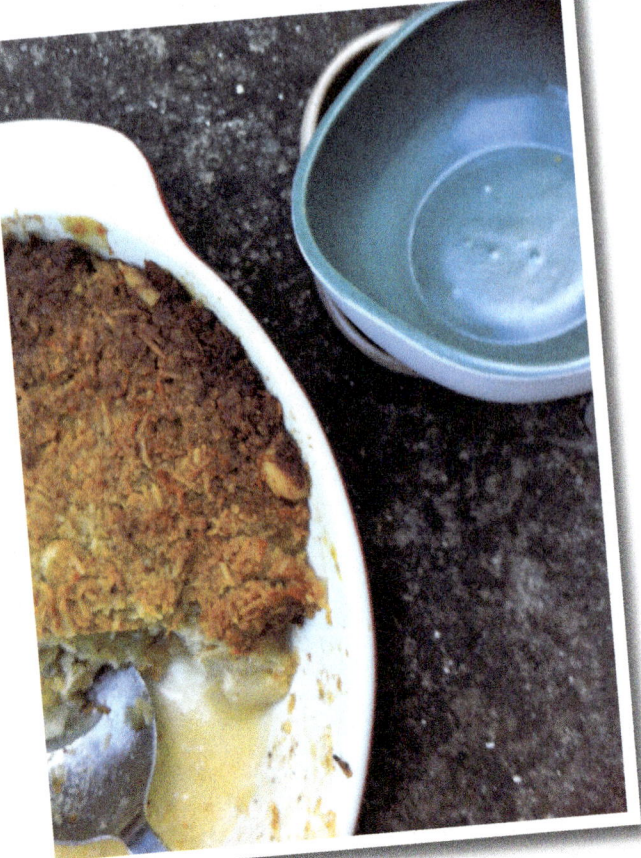

Ingredients

- 6 apples
- 1 orange
- 4 medjool dates
- 150 grams butter or coconut oil
- 1.5 cups desiccated coconut
- 1.5 cups almond flour
- 1 cup walnut or cashews (for a nut free version try ground sunflower seeds)
- 1 tbs raw honey
- Handful of macadamia nuts
- Pinch of salt

To make

1. Peel, core, chop apples.
2. Layer apples and squeeze some orange juice from one orange. Add chopped dates.

Crumble

1. Pre heat oven to 150 degrees C. Take the orange and cut a piece of the peel - do not use any of the white part. Cut finely. Set aside one tbs of the orange skin.
2. Melt butter or coconut oil; add 1.5 cups of desiccated coconut (preservative free) and 1.5 cups of almond flour. Grind one cup of walnut or cashews until in small pieces (use sunflower seeds ground in a coffee grinder if you want a nut free option).
3. Add salt, honey, orange peel and rough chopped macadamia nuts.
4. Mix well in the food processor or with a fork until you have a thick ball.
5. Smooth over the top of your fruit base with the back of a wet tablespoon and put in the oven at 150 degrees for half an hour or until golden brown on top.
6. Serve with your own home made cultured cream.

Apple, orange, macadamia & date crumble.

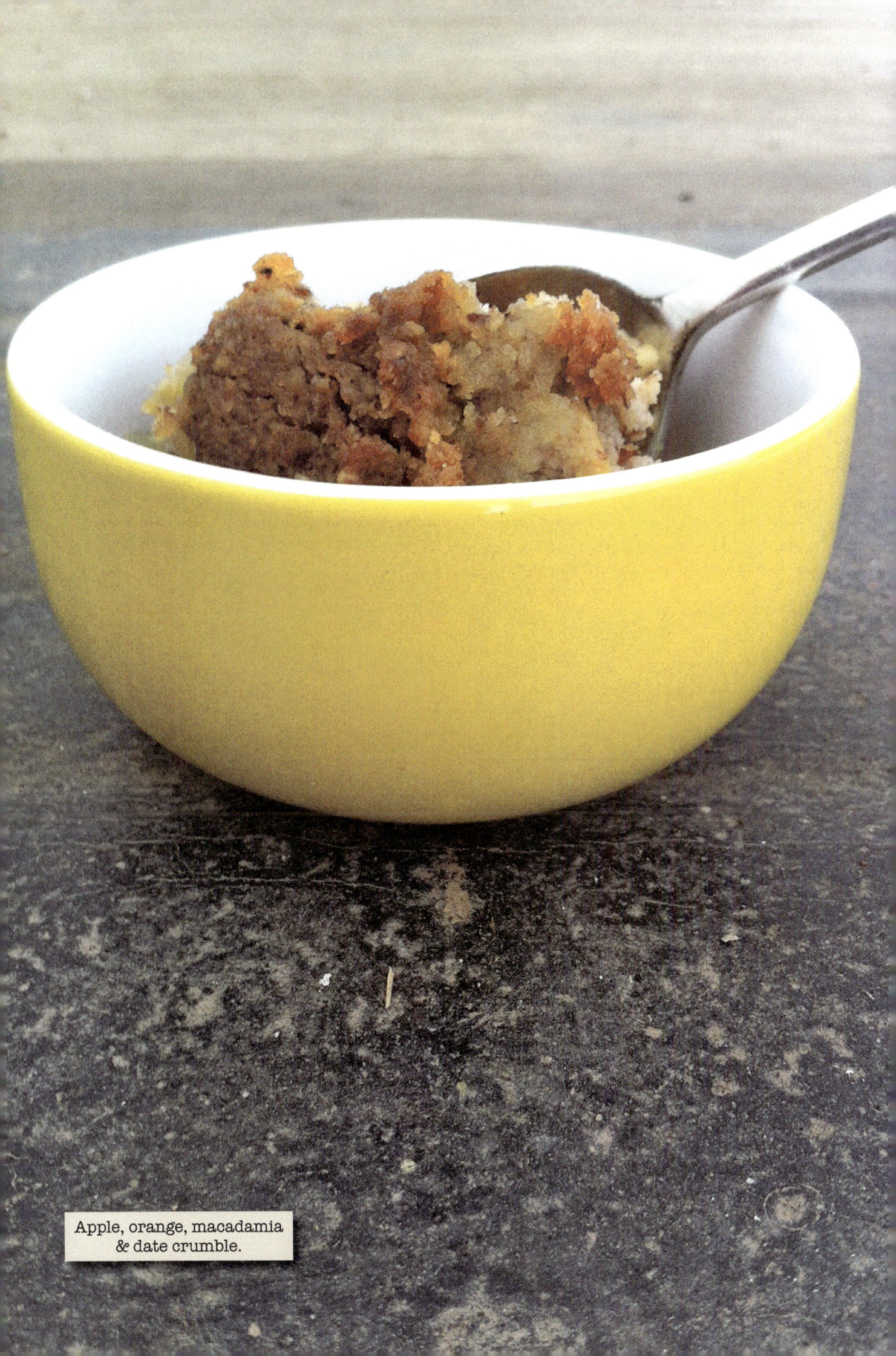

Turkish ginger & apricot cake

It's pretty darn exotic for an allergy friendly cake, I reckon.

This one is egg, nut, dairy (if you want it to be), gluten, grain and sugar free.

> Nuts and seeds can be great but we use them as occasional foods for now.

Nuts and seeds can be hard to digest and you need lots of them to make a cake like this. That's a lot of work for your tum.

My brother's 40th is coming up and we are having a big, fat, family lunch to celebrate. I want something that everyone can enjoy.

For the base

- 1 cup of dried, shredded coconut,
- ½ cup cashews or walnuts
- ½ cup of almonds (nuts soaked overnight makes them more easily digested)
- ½ cup (about 5) pitted Medjool dates
- 2 tbs raw honey (this amps up the sweetness so feel free to scale back if you wish)
- 2 tbs coconut oil

For a nut free option:

- Mix 1½ cups of coconut butter (gently warm on stove till soft)
- ½ cup pitted Medjool dates (about 5 dates).

Note: Bought butters vary, so make sure you like the flavor before making an entire cake with it. Personally, I like the Artisana brand but others make their own at a fraction of the cost with great success. Extra tip: Make friends with someone who has a Thermomix and do a trade.

For the filling

- ½ cup organic dried Turkish apricots sliced finely (dried figs also work beautifully here)
- Two tbs ginger honey - or raw honey if doing GAPS diet
- Six teaspoons Great Lakes Gelatin (get the red one - use only the best quality gelatin. It is full of properties that will help to heal, seal and soothe gut lining). For a veg option, try using agar agar. (N.B. agar is not GAPS appropriate).
- 2 cups cream - Here you can vary. You just need two cups of something.

I did one cup of coconut cream and one cup of thickened dairy cream but you could do all sour cream if you are doing GAPS or all coconut if you have dairy allergy/intolerance.

- ¼ tsp pure vanilla extract or 1 vanilla pod scraped
- ½ teaspoon each of cinnamon, cardamom, ground ginger and nutmeg

Making it

1. Put all the ingredients for the base in the food processor and pulse till bread crumb-like. Line a 9 inch (approx 20cm) cake pan with baking paper and press mix into the base till smooth and flat. Keep the paper in one piece so you can lift it out of the pan. Put in freezer to set.
2. Put apricots on low flame and just cover with water to bring out the sweetness of the apricots. Allow to simmer for a few minutes.
3. Add the gelatine and stir quickly so it dissolves. Allow to cool down to just warm and add the rest of the ingredients and stir until combined. Blend filling with a stick mixer until smooth.
4. Pour the apricot cream into the base, which should be firm. Put the whole lot in the fridge to cool for about 3 hours.
5. Take it out of the fridge half an hour before serving, carefully peel back baking paper. It will be puckered so do it gently.
6. Add more sliced apricots to the top. Drizzle with more honey if you wish. I used some rose petals and calendula.

Extra tip

When using coconut cream I like to use generous amounts of cinnamon, cardamom, ground ginger and nutmeg to help balance its nutty flavour.

Turkish ginger & apricot cake

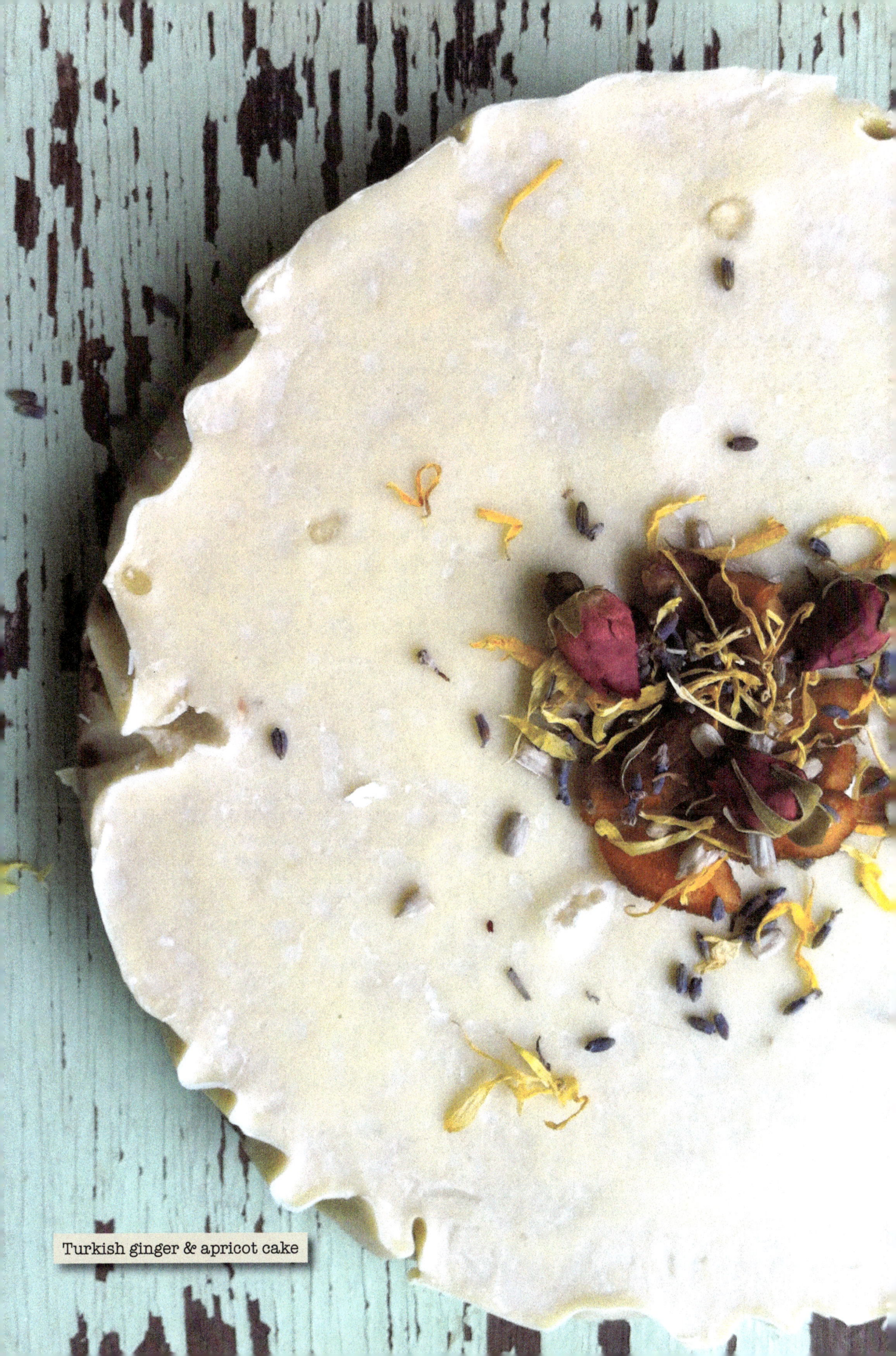

Date & rosewater melting moments

Our children loved these and scoffed them all at once. Lexi, our blue heeler, kelpie cross darted around our feet licking crumbs off our toes and the floor.

James and I loved them too. The date filling is incredible.

The real test will be to offer them to some little friends as the texture is different to store bought biscuits. However, for us, a double batch will be necessary next time I think.

Make them as melting moments or use the filling as an icing on top of one single biscuit.

Feel free to add a little bit of cocoa powder if you fancy something chocolatey.

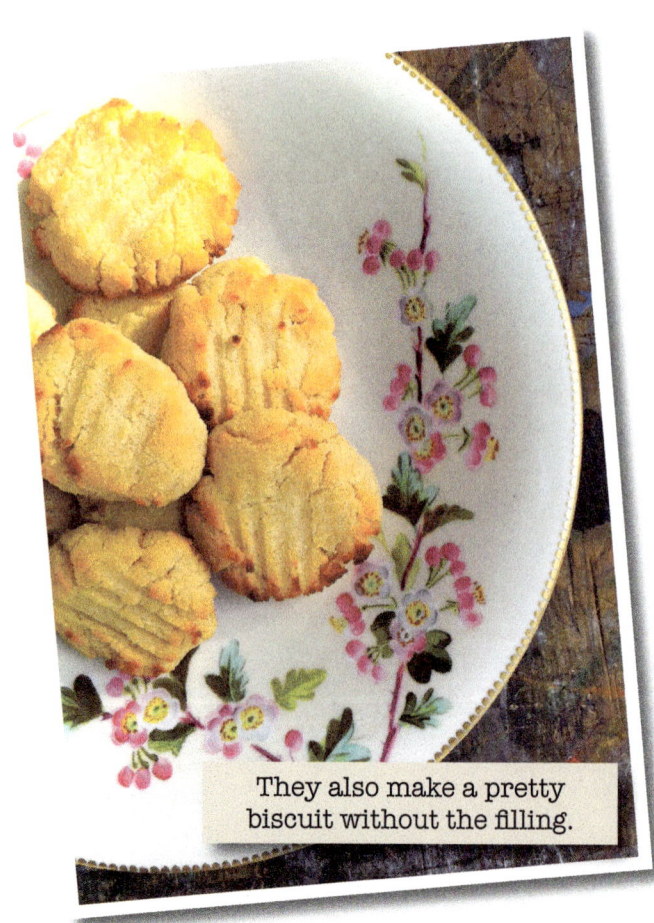

They also make a pretty biscuit without the filling.

Ingredients

Biscuits

- ½ cup coconut flour
- 150 grams of butter (or coconut oil or macadamia nut oil)
- 1 tsp vanilla extract
- pinch of salt
- 2 tsp of rosewater
- 2 tablespoons of raw honey
- 1 tablespoon of finely chopped organic orange rind
- 1 tsp gelatine dissolved in 2 tablespoons of hot water

Date filling

Two dates soaked in a little warm water for five minutes until soft, blend until smooth and you have a thick paste.

Making it

1. Preheat oven to 180 degrees C.
2. Melt butter on the stove and add wet ingredients to saucepan to dissolve.
3. Add this to the coconut flour and salt. Mix well and roll into small balls on baking paper. These will not spread or change shape.
4. Flatten with a fork and reshape biscuits into rounds if they begin to lose their shape.
5. Bake for about 10 minutes or until golden. Wait until biscuits are cool before you handle them as they will crumble before the gelatine gets a chance to do its work holding them together.
6. As the biscuits cool, take two tablespoons of coconut butter in a small bowl (I like the Artisana brand best) and mix in dates. Add a teaspoon of rosewater and mix to a smooth paste.
7. Spoon the filling on the underside of a biscuit and put another on top.

Extra tip

Use this date filling between any homemade biscuits you like. They are great with the cookies featured on page 104.

Date & rosewater
melting moments.

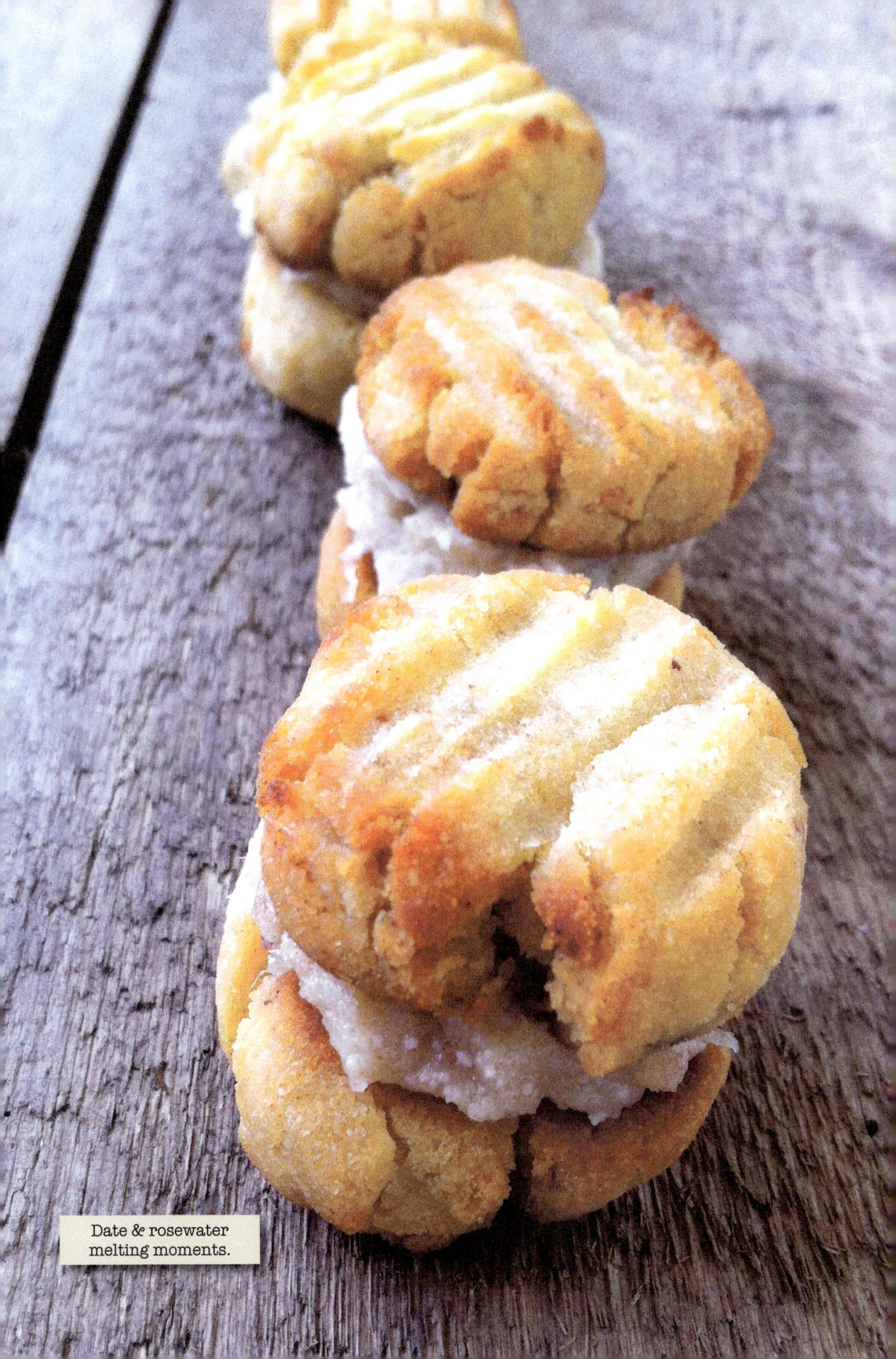

Instant chocolate raspberry ice cream

This egg free, dairy free dessert has a smooth and creamy quality to it. It's the one that gets wow factor every time I serve it. Friends always ask for the recipe.

It works well as a very quick-to-make ice cream or a decadent chocolate mousse. It is also delicious as a pie or tart filler.

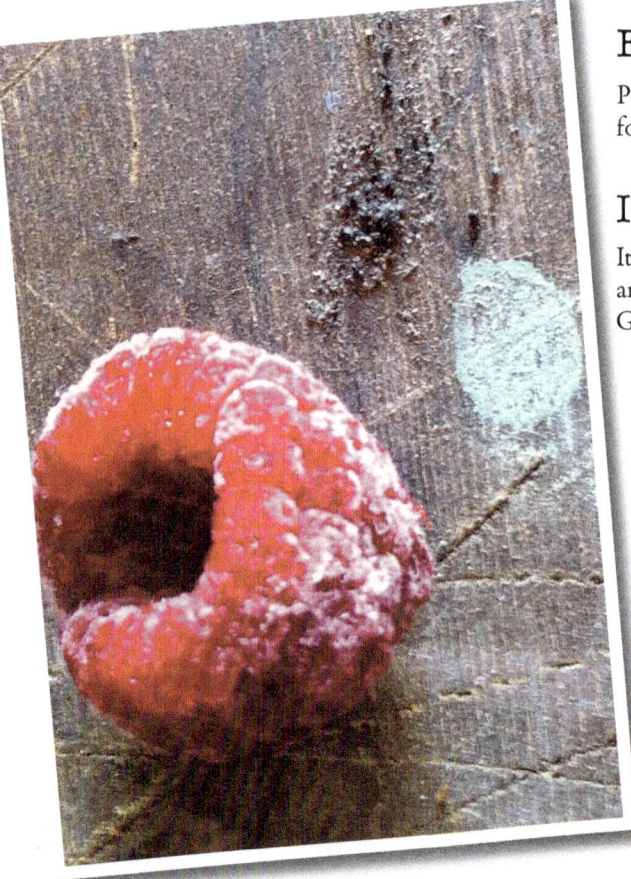

Ingredients

- 1 quarter avocado
- 1 frozen banana
- 4 dates chopped
- 1 cup frozen raspberries (I only use organic when it comes to berries)
- Pinch of salt (this helps to balance the flavours)
- 1 teaspoon of vanilla extract or one vanilla pod scraped
- 2 tablespoons of cocoa (add gradually & to taste)

Making it

1. Whizz it all together in a food processor until smooth. Stir through a few more fresh raspberries for texture.
2. You could also mix in some home made marshmallows for an extra treat. Add raw honey if desired.
3. Keep in the freezer and take out about 20 minutes before serving so the ice cream is frozen but soft enough to put a spoon through.

Extra tip

Peel bananas and avocados, cut them into pieces and freeze for future use.

Important note

It is advised to hold off on chocolate until a considerable amount of healing has been done if you are following the GAPS Diet.

Instant chocolate raspberry ice cream

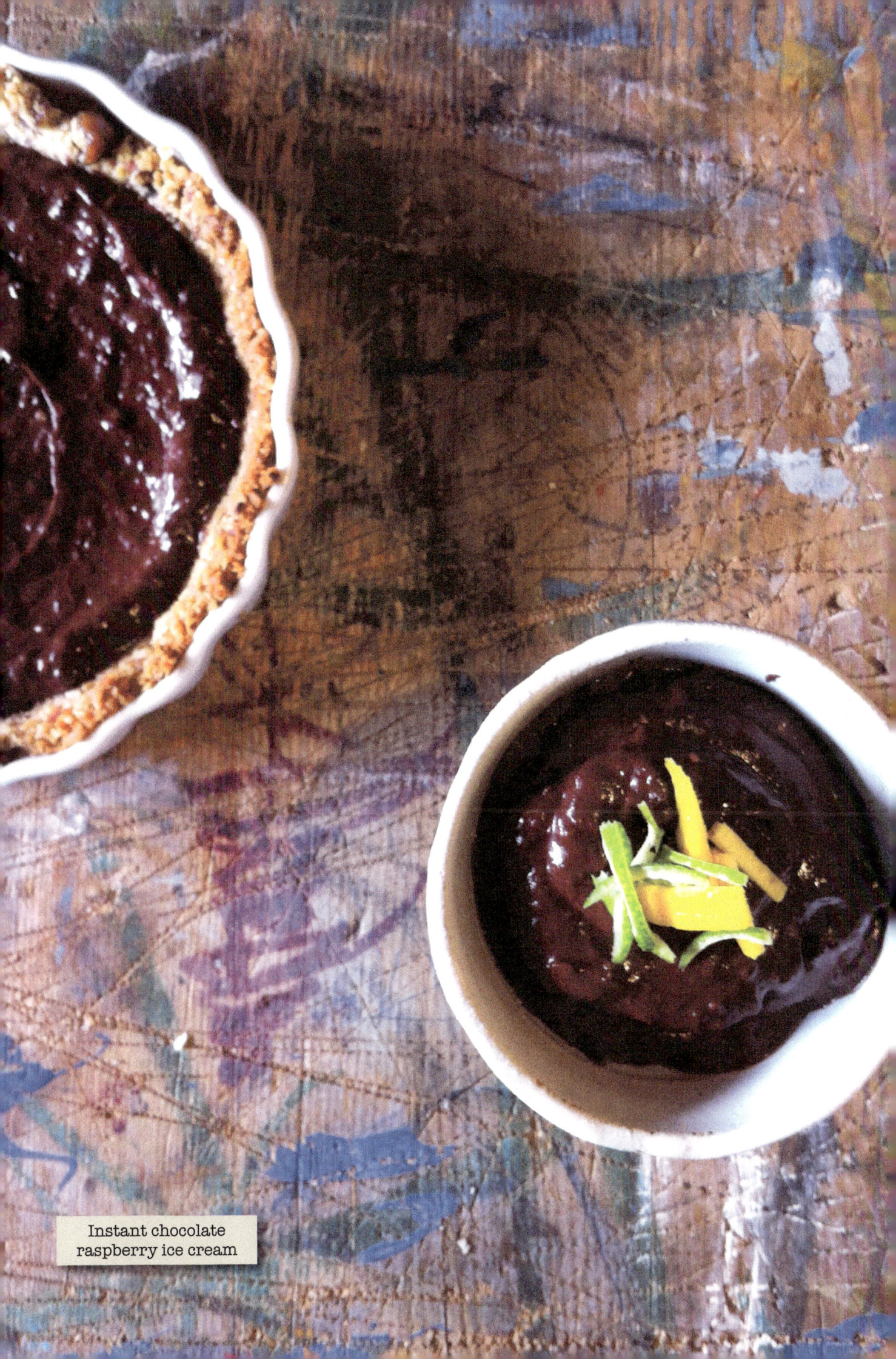

Mixed berry mousse

We are so lucky living where we do.

The Bellarine Peninsula is packed with local producers doing amazing things.

About 15 minutes down the road is Tuckerberry Hill Farm where you can pick your own strawberries and blueberries when they are in season.

A major plus is that on the weekend the farm also plays host to the Buy Bellarine Produce Barn where local producers gather their freshest, most delicious goodies and sell it all under one roof.

There's local honey, olive oil, sourdough bread, organic and conventional veggies, seeds, cheeses, meats, the list goes on and on.

> We went home and made what I have called mixed berry mousse. It is egg free and is actually a variation on our ice cream but my kids and I could not stand the wait.

Ingredients

- Half a ripe avocado
- 1 ripe banana
- 1 punnet of strawberries
- 1 cup of blueberries (I had frozen ones from last year's blueberry season at Tuckerberry Hill)
- 6 medjool dates (seeds removed) and chop finely
- 1 cup of cultured cream or coconut milk
- 2 tsp gelatine
- Pinch of salt

Making it

1. Dissolve gelatine into two tbs of boiling water. Stir quickly until all grains are disolved
2. Whizz all ingredients up in a food processor and spoon into something pretty.
3. Allow to set in the fridge for about half an hour.

Extra Tip

I sometimes give these to our girls as a brekky treat in the summertime.

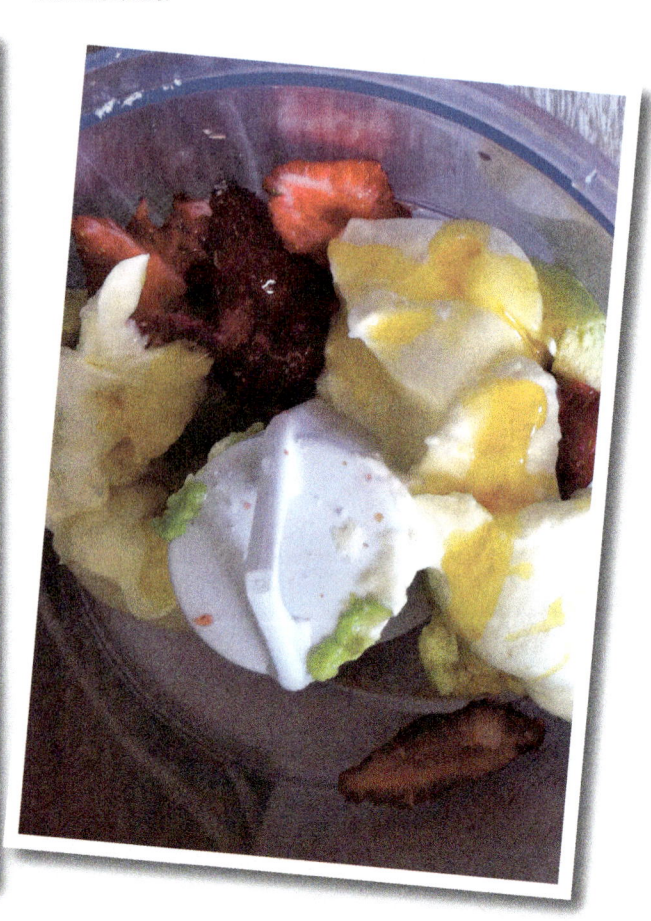

Bike snacks.

Mixed Berry Mousse

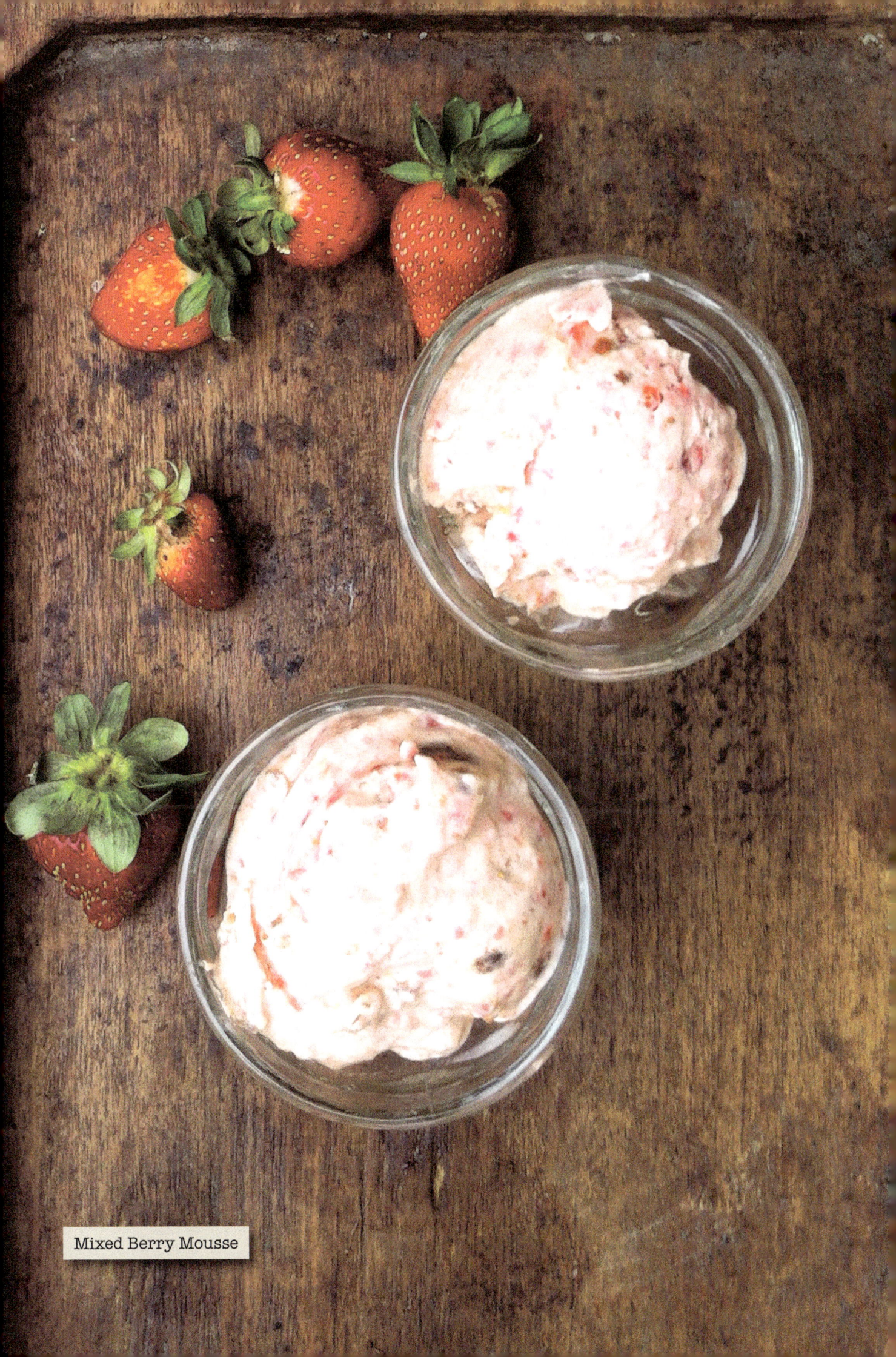

Raw honey panna cotta with vanilla & orange extract

This is a simple and elegant dessert that you can make in minutes.

It serves well as an after kinder/school snack on a hot day and makes an easy cross-over to a more grown-up dinner party. I love that it is rich in natural probiotics as I have used cultured cream, however, you could also use coconut milk if you wanted to do a dairy free version.

I choose to sweeten with raw honey in my recipes as it is more easily digested, is an antiseptic, and provides vitamins and minerals.

Traditionally it has been used to treat digestive disorders, as well as chest and throat infections. If using cultured cream, this dessert, combined with the gut healing properties of gelatine can make for a very soothing treat.

Many leave out the fruit until a significant amount of gut healing has taken place, preferring to stick to simple stocks, stews, cultured dairy such as yoghurt and cream and cultured vegetables.

> When it comes to honey, I find just the tiniest amount is enough for a young palate and please be aware of the risks of serving honey to a very small child under 12 months.

Cooking Note: Be sure to dissolve the gelatine in hot water and whisk quickly before adding the cultured cream.

I allow the gelatine mix to be luke warm, so as not to kill the beneficial bacteria in the cream.

I created this serve for our two little girls, but you could easily double the proportions for more people - or even better - make a large batch to last you a few days.

It also makes a great no-cook pie filling.

Think, gluten, grain, sugar free base as per the Turkish apricot cake, panna cotta filling, fresh berries on top.

Amazing!

Ingredients

- 3 tsp Great Lakes Gelatin (or any other gelatine that is from grass fed bovines)
- ¼ cup boiled, filtered water
- 1 cup cultured cream, milk kefir or coconut milk
- 1 teaspoon vanilla and orange extract or 1 scraped vanilla pod
- 1 tsp raw honey (or to taste)

Making it

1. Dissolve the gelatine in a bowl of boiled water whisking immediately and continuously.
2. When gelatine mix is luke warm, quickly whisk in cultured cream
3. Add raw honey and vanilla orange extract and whisk until completely smooth.
4. Pour into ramekins or anything pretty you know your children will love.
5. If using ramekins, dip them in warm water for a few minutes and turn them out onto a cold plate to serve.
6. Serve with whatever seasonal fruit you have at home. Berries are a favourite in summer but try oven roasted peaches or poached pears with ginger and turmeric in winter months.

Extra tip

Change up the flavours of the panna cotta by making the most of spices.

Try a chai spiced panna cotta by adding 1 tsp of ground cinnamon, cardamom, ginger and nutmeg to the vanilla extract. So yum.

Add a little cocoa to make a chocolate treat. I do about a tablespoon of cocoa to a cup of cream. Cinnamon and ginger are also great additions here.

A beautiful *non dairy* summery panna cotta is made by blending up your cup of coconut milk with two mango cheeks and a really good squeeze of lime. Also try pineapple or papaya and fresh mint.

The options are endless.

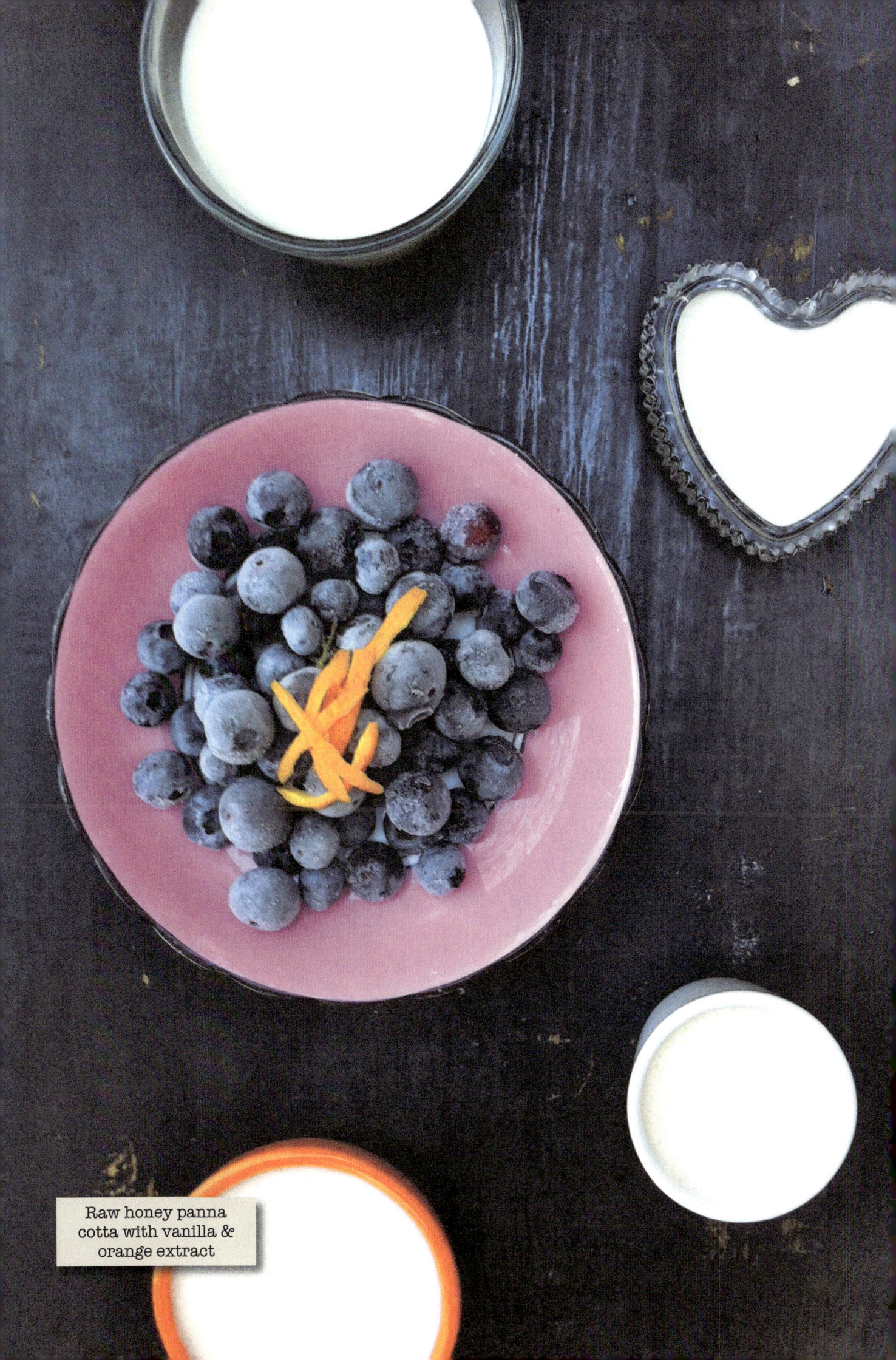

Raw honey panna cotta with vanilla & orange extract

Poached pears in turmeric & ginger

This is a beautiful little Autumn breakfast dish when pears have just come into season and the mornings start fresh and become bright, clear and sunny.

Turmeric is a great immune system booster.

Ginger is warming and very supportive to the digestive system.

I often cook these when someone in our family has a cold. It is sweet, soothing and comforting as well as being a gentle way to start the day.

Making it

1. Peel the skin of four pears and cut into thick slices.
2. Cut about a thumb-sized piece of ginger and turmeric thickly into slices.
3. Cover the pears with a good amount of water and poach gently with the lid on for about 30 mins.
4. Serve warm with a dollop of your favourite home made yoghurt.

Extra tip

I often poach in the evening and allow the flavours to meld overnight.

Reserve pear juice and use for smoothies, jellies or icy poles.

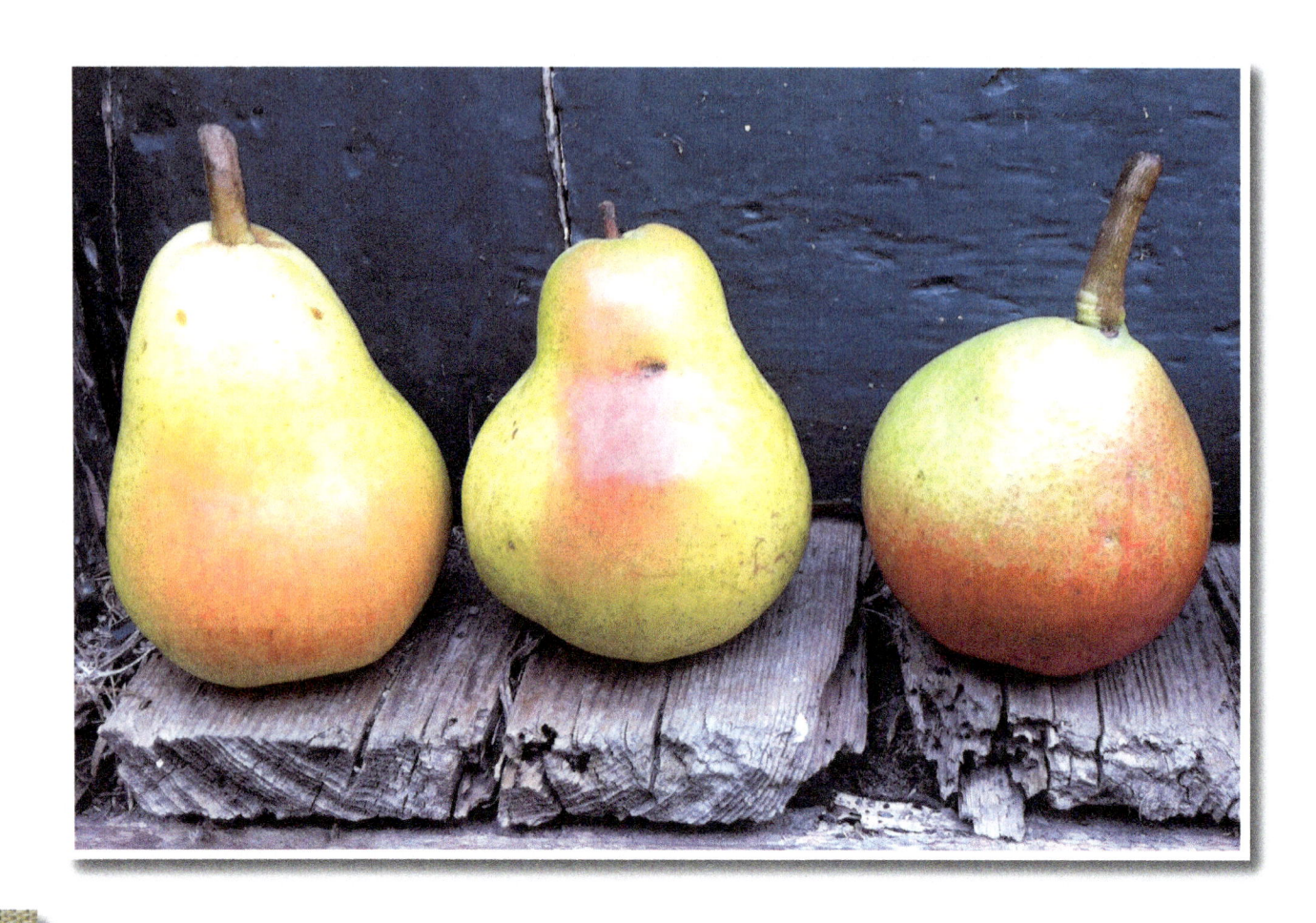

Poached pears with tumeric and ginger.

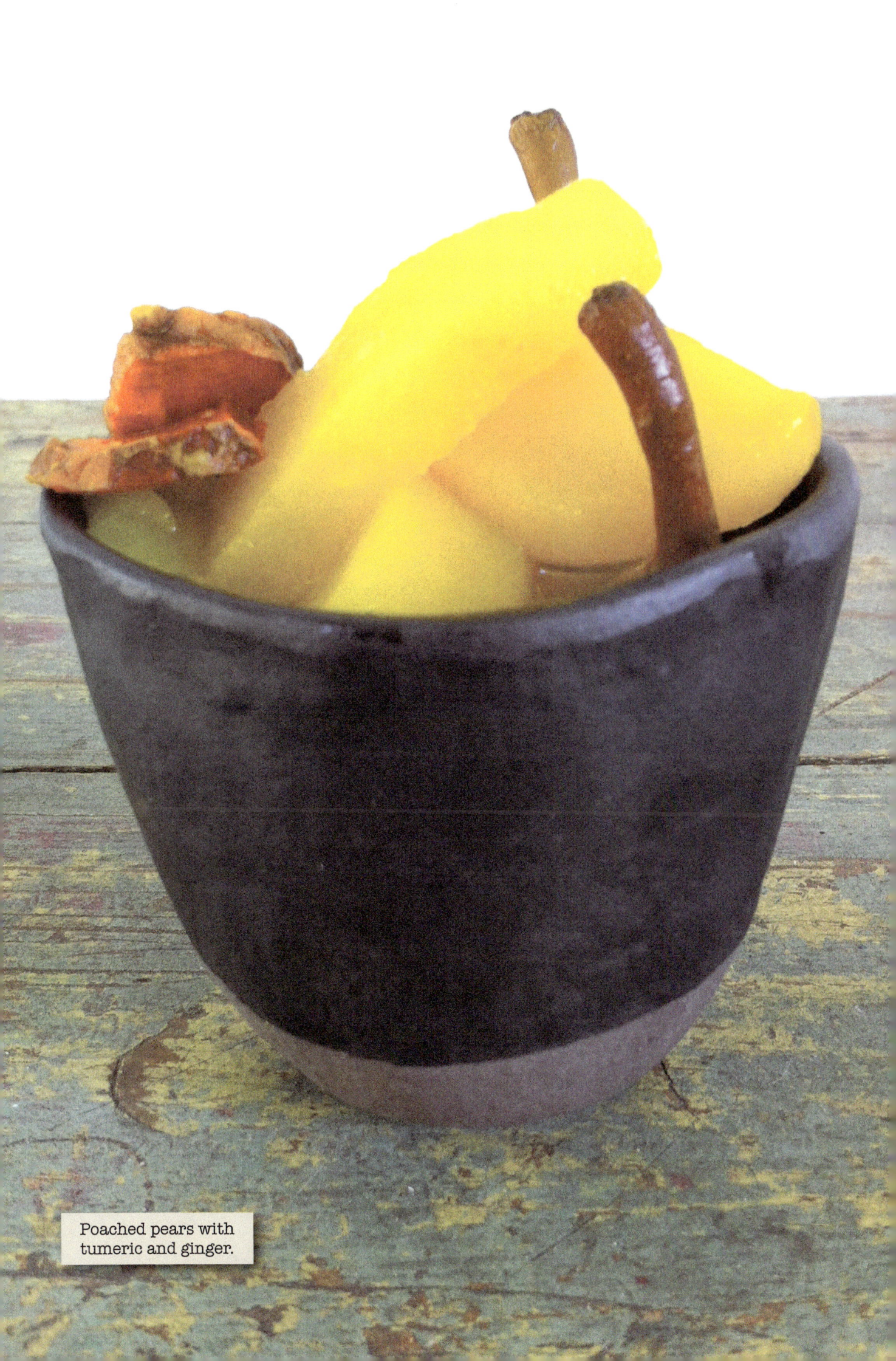

Gluten & grain free cookies

These take no time at all.

If you need to be nut free for school or allergies, sub the almond meal with sunflower seeds ground in a coffee grinder.

This also makes a great base for a sweet tart or cake.

Ingredients

- 100 grams of butter or coconut oil
- 1 cup almond meal, (or a mix of finely ground pumpkin and sunflower seeds)
- 1 tbs raw honey
- 1 pinch salt

Optional: Cocoa, dried apricots, dates and/or figs, macadamia nuts (for an extra flavour boost soak the dried fruits in some melted butter).

Making it

1. Put ingredients in a food processor and whizz till everything comes together.
2. Turn out onto a piece of baking paper and use the paper to roll into a log.
3. Put into the freezer for about 15 mins to chill. This will make cutting the cookies easier. (this step is optional)
4. Unroll the baking paper and cut into two cm rounds.
5. Bake until golden on 150 deg C for about 30 minutes depending on your oven.

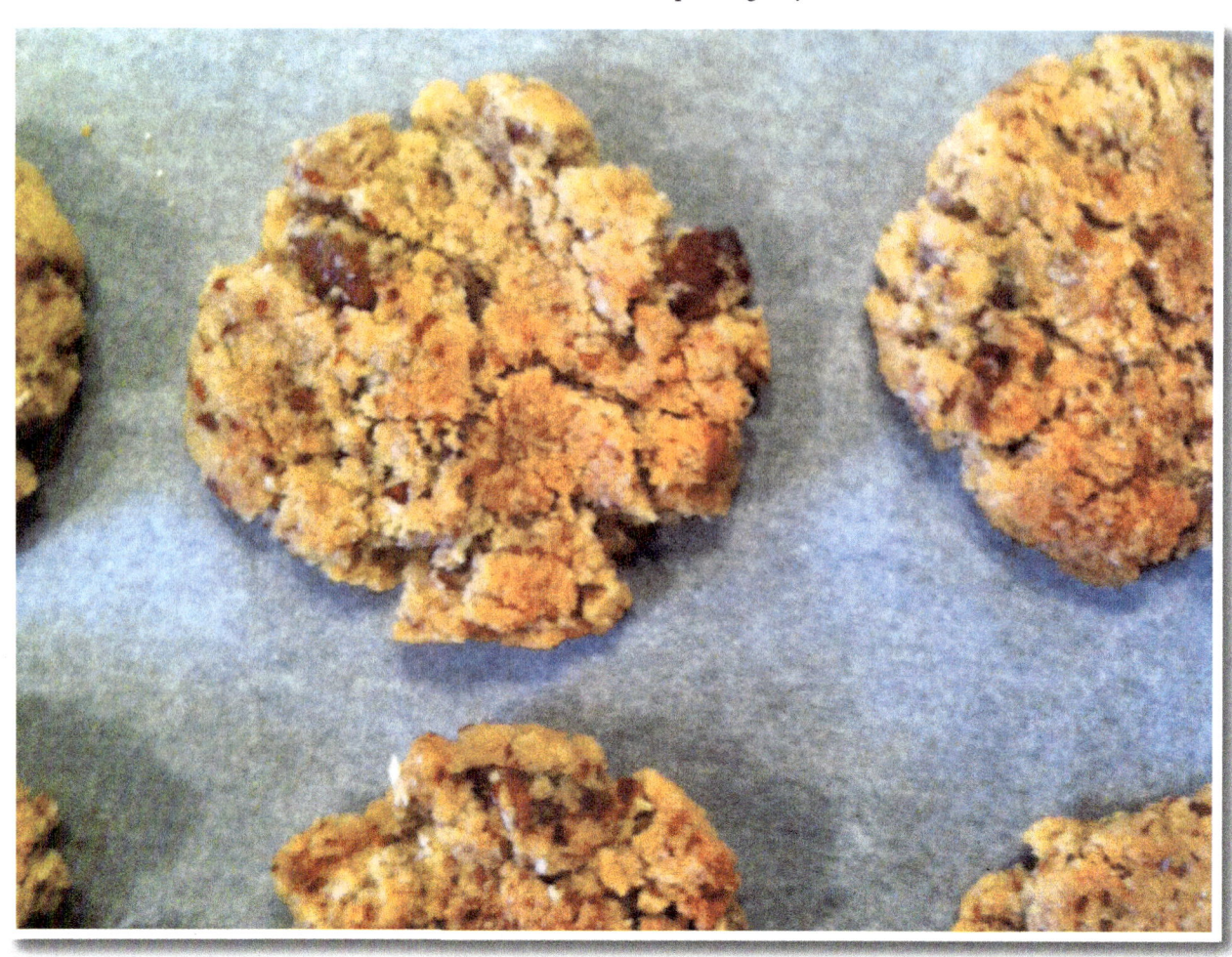

Two-minute cultured raspberry ice cream

When the first of the raspberries come in we make the most of them.

Plump, sweet and sour, these hairy little jewels are amazing.

This is a lovely little warm weather treat if you don't want to use any eggs, heat or sweetener. Feel free to substitute with any other berry you love and is in season.

Making it

1. In the food processor I whizzed approximately half a punnet of raspberries, together with a quarter of an avocado, half a ripe banana and some of our home made cultured cream. (for a dairy free option use coconut milk or coconut cream)

2. You could also add a pinch of good salt and some vanilla bean scraped in if you wanted.

3. Put into little ice cream moulds (We got ours from the $2 shop).

4. Ours set in a couple of hours. Run it under water at first to let the ice cream loosen and gently pull it from the mould.

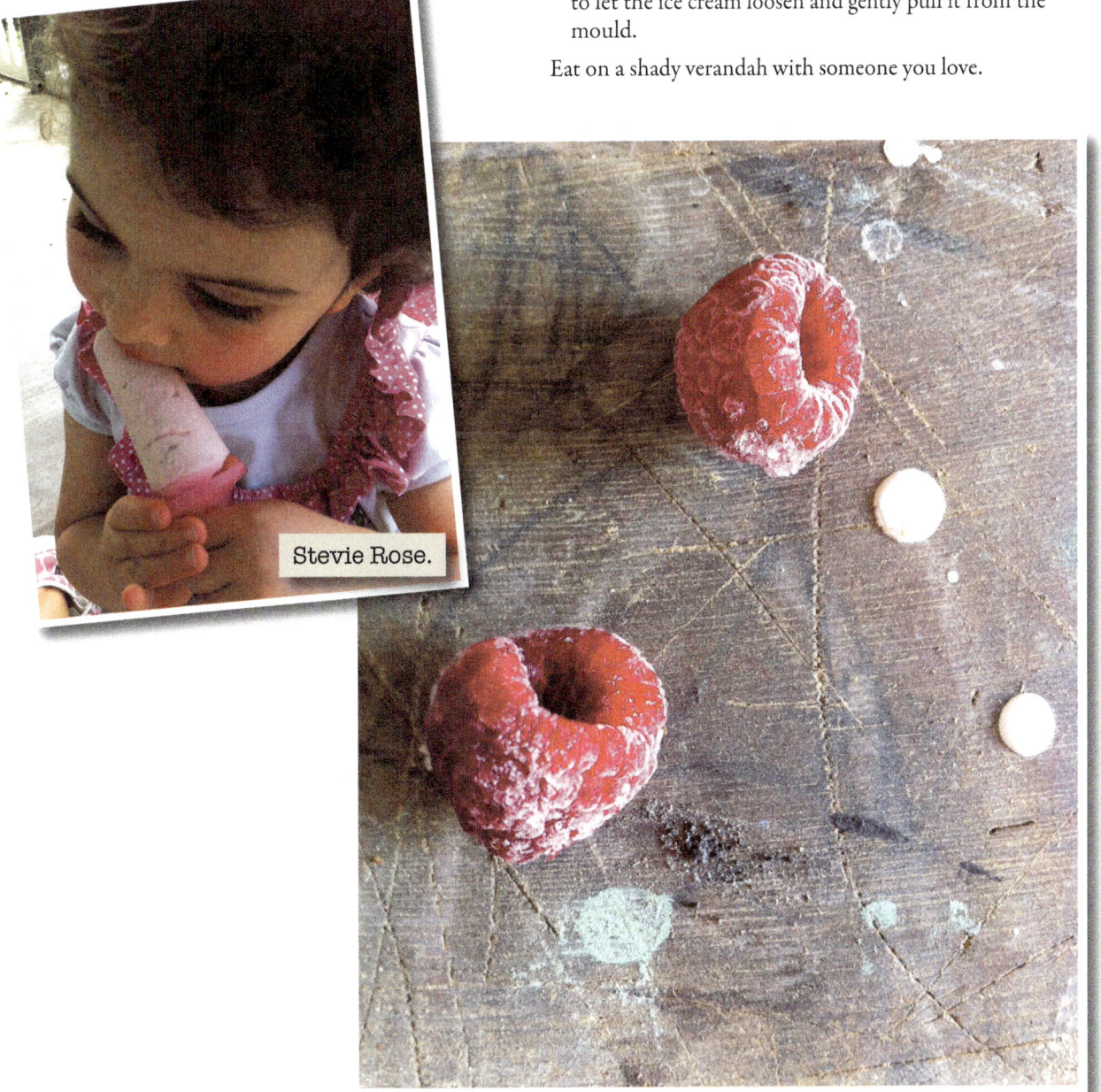

Eat on a shady verandah with someone you love.

Stevie Rose.

Egyptian rosewater honey cake

Another gluten free, grain free, sugar free adaption.

This one is thanks to my grandmother Dianne.

Born in Alexandria, her classic migrant journey paved the way for me to live this fortunate life here in this little village by the sea.

Many thanks to you Nanni. Our culture travels the generations as we grow and change as we must.

We call this one *Harissa* at home and it is a family favourite.

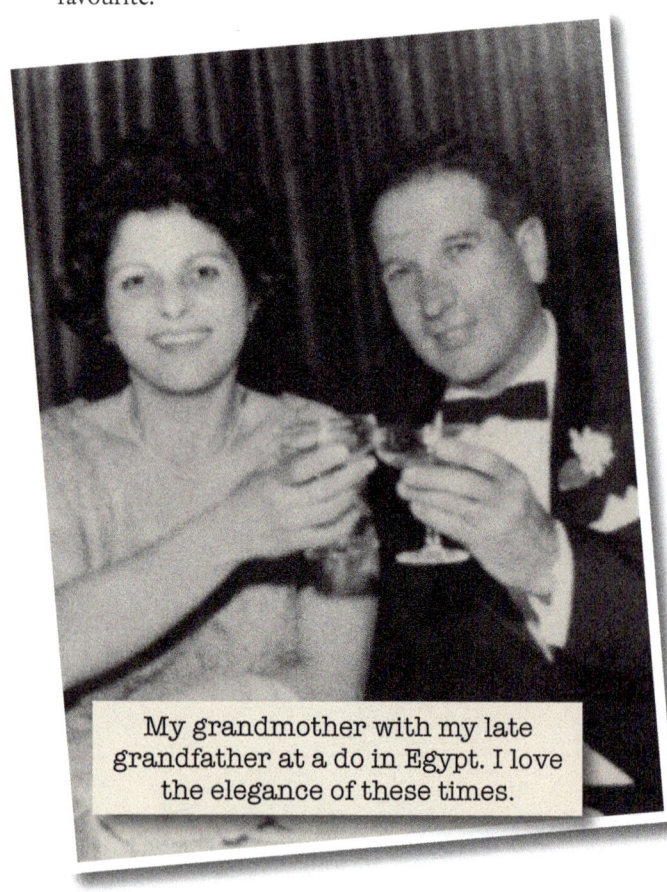

My grandmother with my late grandfather at a do in Egypt. I love the elegance of these times.

Nanni is a pocket rocket and going strong but has sadly retired from the kitchen. Harissa is my job now. Still, I can't eat this dessert ever without thinking about the way she would proudly and delightedly present it to us in a big tray at family celebrations. We would all insist in advance that she make it.

Rosewater syrup

- 1 cup water
- ½ cup raw honey
- 1 ½ tablespoons lemon juice
- 1 teaspoon rosewater

Making it

1. Combine water and honey in a small saucepan
2. Bring to the boil and then simmer until syrupy, about five minutes.
3. Stir in lemon juice and rosewater
4. Allow to cool completely.

Cake

- 100 grams of butter
- 1 cup desiccated coconut
- ½ cup cashew meal
- 1 cup almond meal (traditionally semolina is used)
- 1 pinch salt

Making it

1. Mix all together in a food processor.
2. Turn out into a small baking dish
3. Smooth down with a wet tablespoon
4. Use a very sharp knife to cut serrations on the diagonal, then cut again on the other diagonal until you have a series of diamond shapes.
5. Bake at 150 degrees C for about half an hour or until golden brown.
6. Gently pour cool syrup on to the warm cake. Allow it to soak in.
7. If there is too much liquid put dish back into the oven to bake some more.
8. Otherwise leave for about half an hour.
9. Serve with cultured cream or yoghurt, fresh pomegranate and mint leaves.

Egyptian rosewater honey cake.

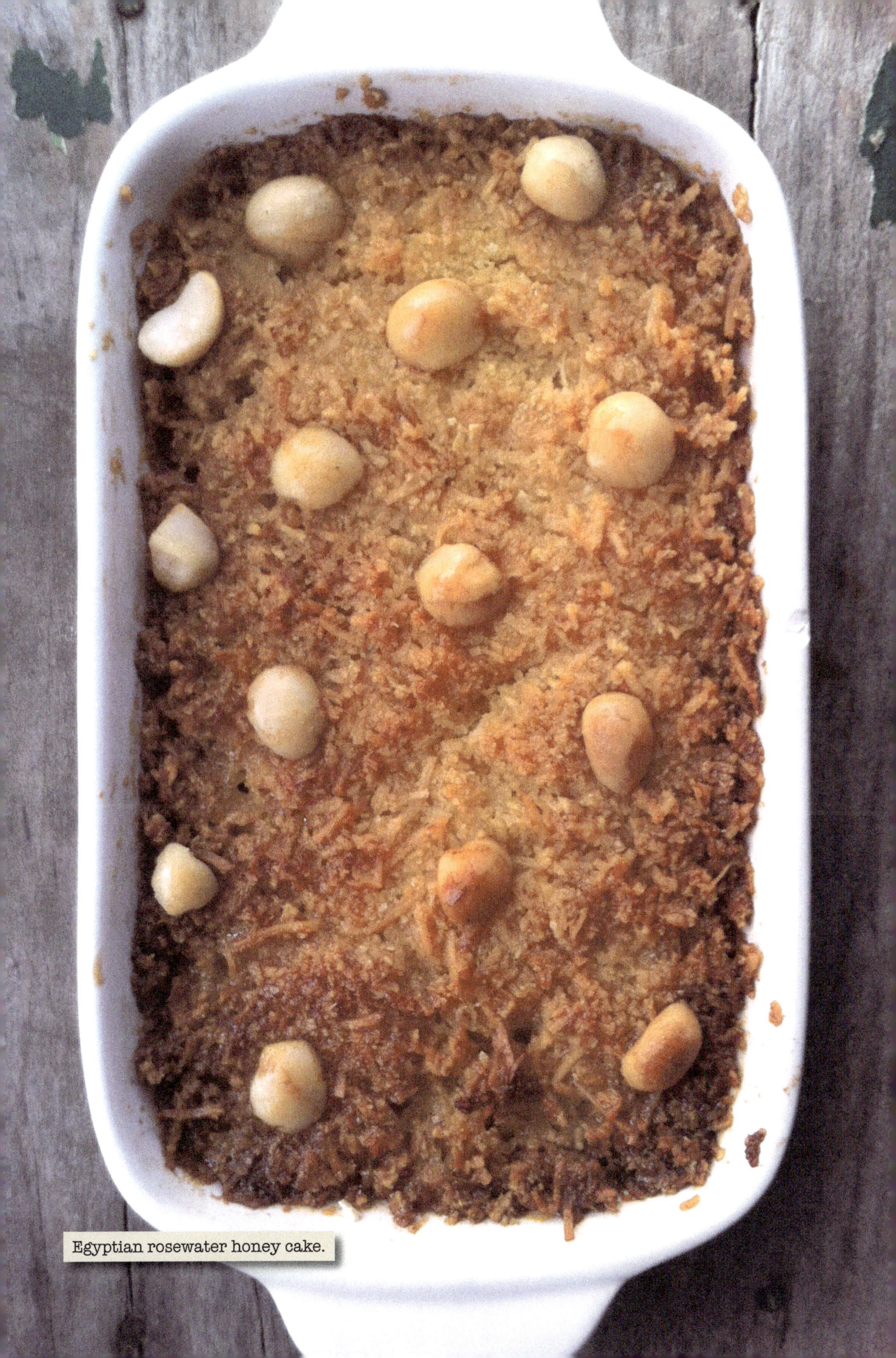

Orange blossom blueberry pie

Gluten free, grain free, refined sugar free. This is a sweet little baby cake.

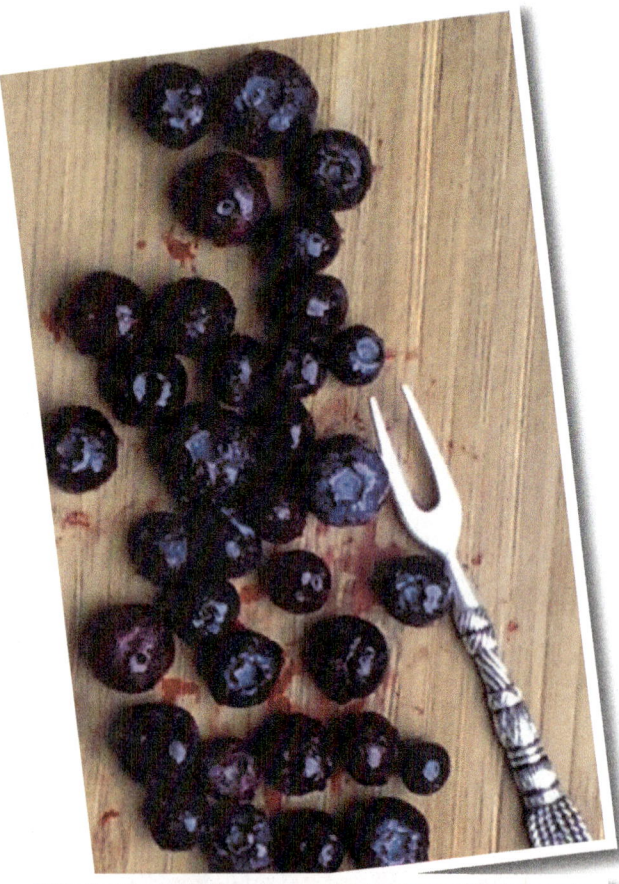

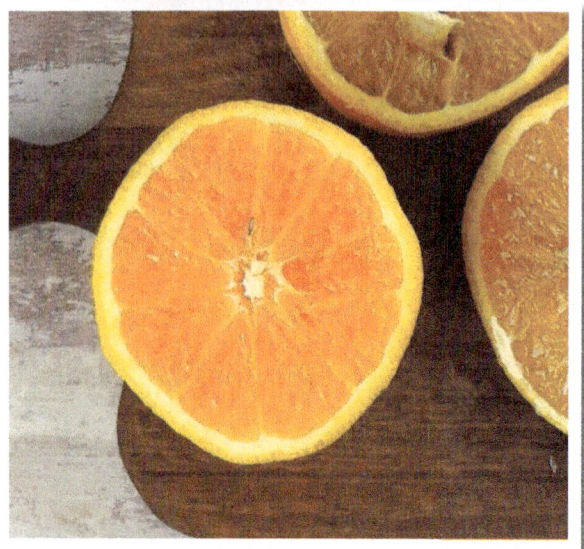

Base

- 100 grams of butter
- 1 cup desiccated coconut
- ½ cup cashew meal
- ½ cup almond meal or sunflower seeds for a nut free option
- 1 pinch salt
- tbs raw honey
- 5 medjool dates, chopped

Making it

1. Blend the ingredients in a food processor, take the mixture and press it into small, individual ceramic pie dishes with your fingers.

Filling

- 1 tbs of raw honey
- 1 cup of yoghurt or coconut cream (for a dairy free option)
- 2 tbs cultured cream if using dairy
- 3 tsp of gelatine dissolved in boiling water
- orange blossom raw honey to drizzle on top
- 1 scraped vanilla pod

Making it

1. Blend the base ingredients in a food processor , take the mixture and press it into a small, individual ceramic pie dishes with your fingers.
2. Bake it in the oven at 150 degrees Celsius for 30 minutes or until golden.
3. Allow to cool.
4. With a hand mixer, blend one cup of yoghurt with two tablespoons of cultured cream. You should have a nice thick mixture. (For variety add ½ a cup of any kind of fruit you wish here. The options are endless.)
5. Blend the filling ingredients with the gelatine
6. Spoon into cooled tart case and drizzle with raw honey – used one flavoured with orange blossom for this one.
7. Allow to set in the fridge for about half an hour
8. Top with seasonal berries or sliced fruit of any kind. You could even top with pan fried nectarines, or burnt butter pears.

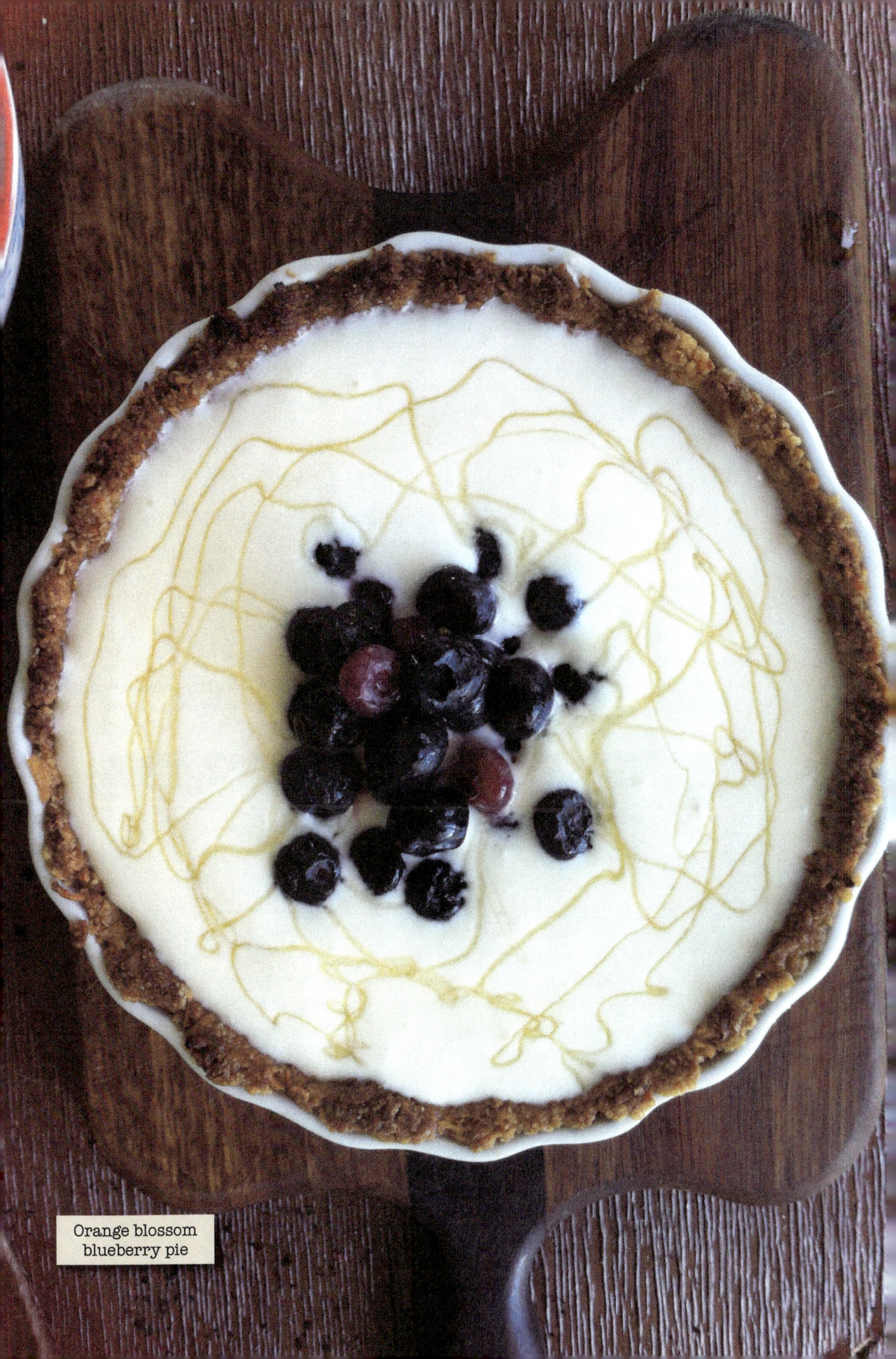

Orange blossom blueberry pie

Banana cream brekky custards

This little treat is a perfect way to warm up on a cold morning.

Prepare in advance and reheat or whizz it up and put it in the oven first thing.

Your whole house will smell deliciously of banana and vanilla. Yum. It's also egg and dairy free.

Ingredients

- 2 ripe bananas chopped roughly
- 1 cup coconut cream
- 1 vanilla pod, scraped
- Pinch of salt
- 2 tsp of gelatine, dissolved in 1 tbs of warm water
- 1 teaspoon of raw honey (add more as desired)
- 1 teaspoon of cinnamon, ground
- ½ teaspoon of ginger, ground
- ½ teaspoon of cardamom, ground

Making it

1. Blend together with a stick mixer and pour into ramekins.
2. Sprinkle with cinnamon and bake at 180 degrees C for about 30 minutes, or until golden brown.

Extra tip

Now that we can have eggs, I have been including them in this recipe with beautiful results. Whisk four eggs to this list of ingredients for an even more decadent custard.

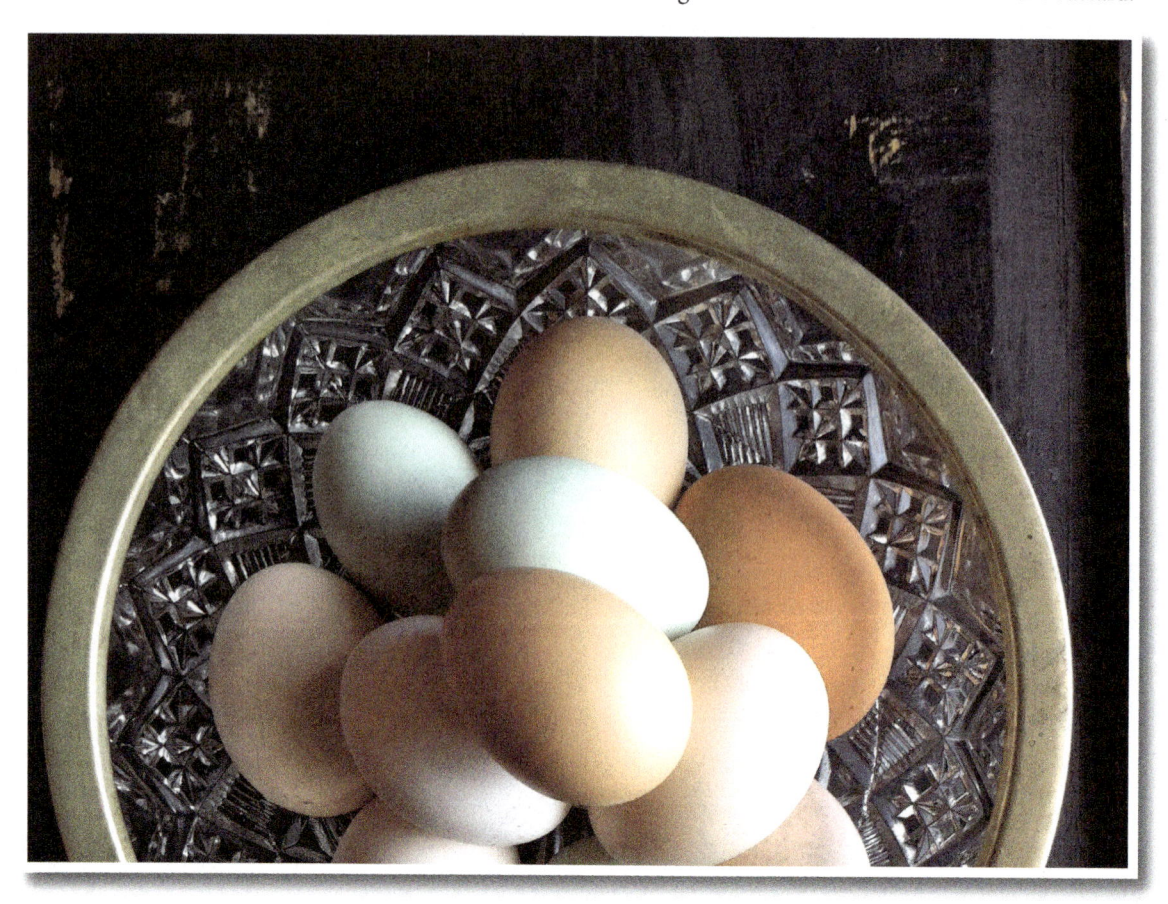

Banana cream brekky custards.

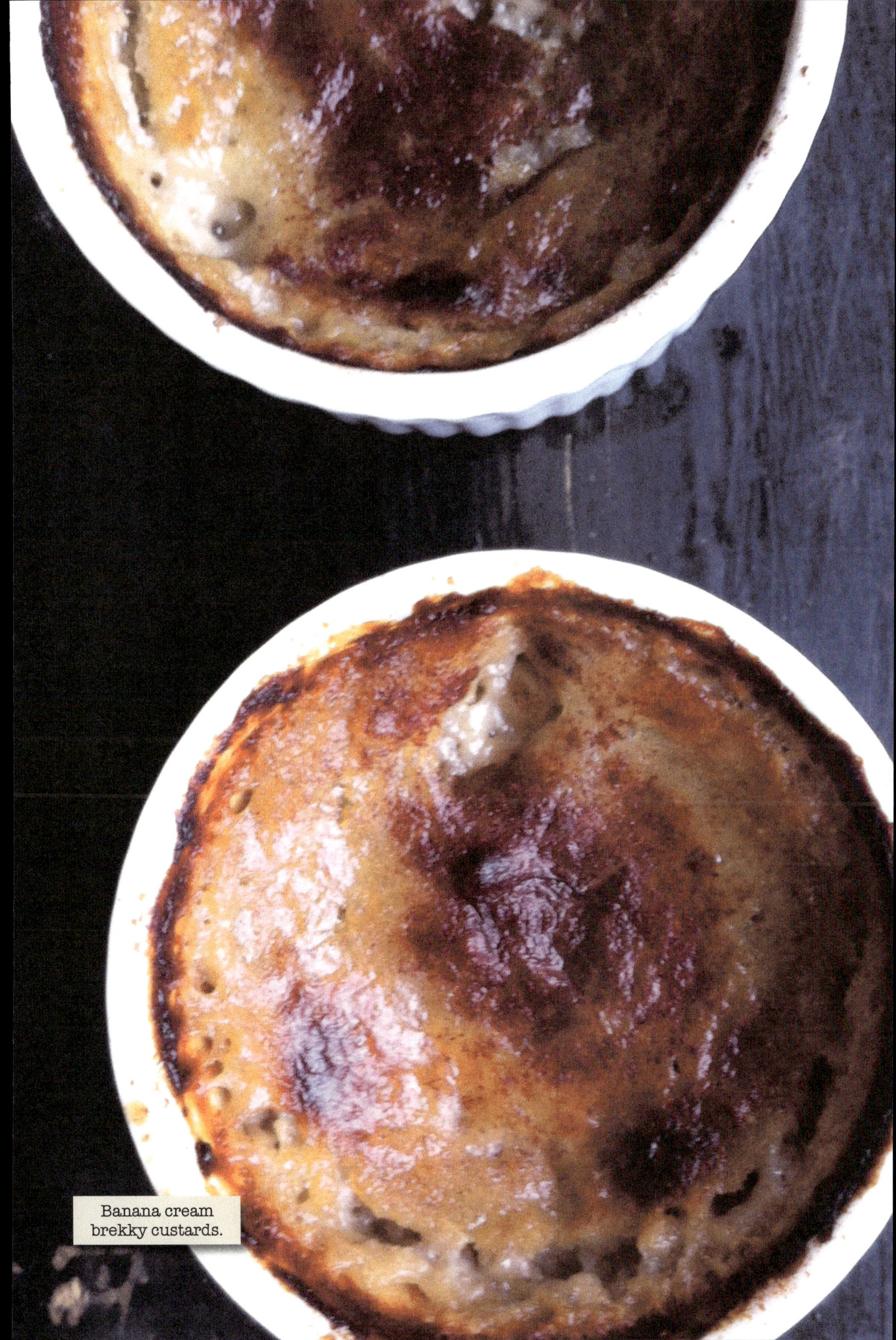

Tropical coconut, mango, passionfruit creams

Another very quick and simple recipe using all the best ingredients summer has to offer.

Coconut milk goes very well with mango and passionfruit. I love to add a bit of ginger for extra tropical kick. Lime or lemon juice also lend a tartness to the dessert that I love. Dairy free tropical mango and passionfruit creams.

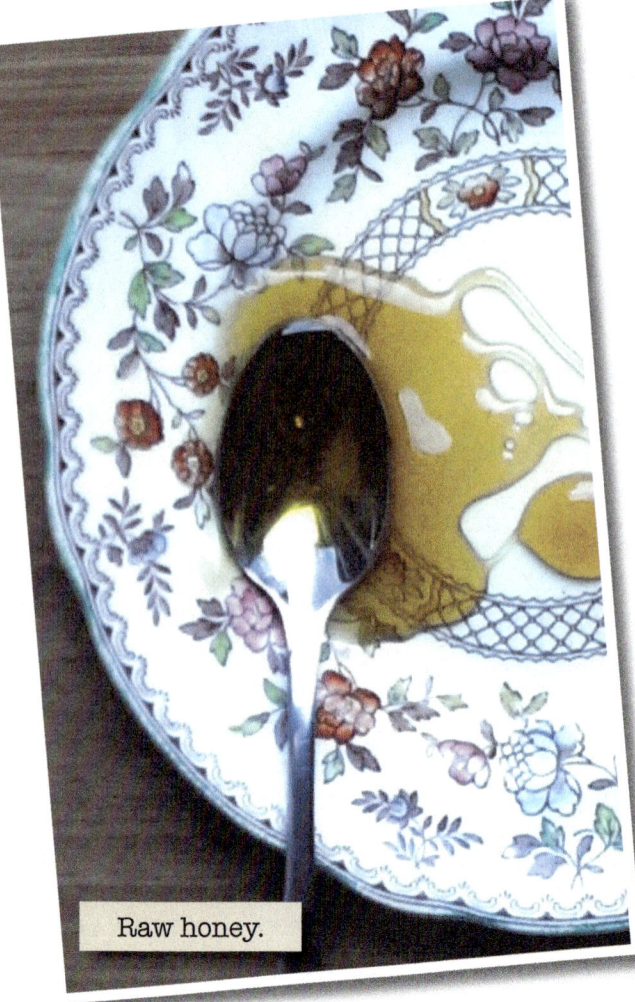

Ingredients

- 1 cup of the best quality, organic, BPA free coconut milk you can find (or even better, make it yourself).
- 1 tablespoon raw ginger honey
- 2 mango cheeks, diced
- Pulp of one passionfruit
- 1 vanilla bean, scraped
- 2 teaspoons of the red Great Lakes Gelatin dissolved in 1 tbs of hot water.
- Squeeze of lemon or lime (about a teaspoon).

Making it

1. Whizz all ingredients except the passionfruit with a stick mixer until smooth.
2. Stir through half the passionfruit pulp and pour into individual ramekins.
3. Refrigerate until firm. Should take about one hour max.
4. Serve with the rest of the passionfruit pulp on top, together with some zested lime for garnish.

Raw honey.

Tropical coconut, mango, passionfruit creams

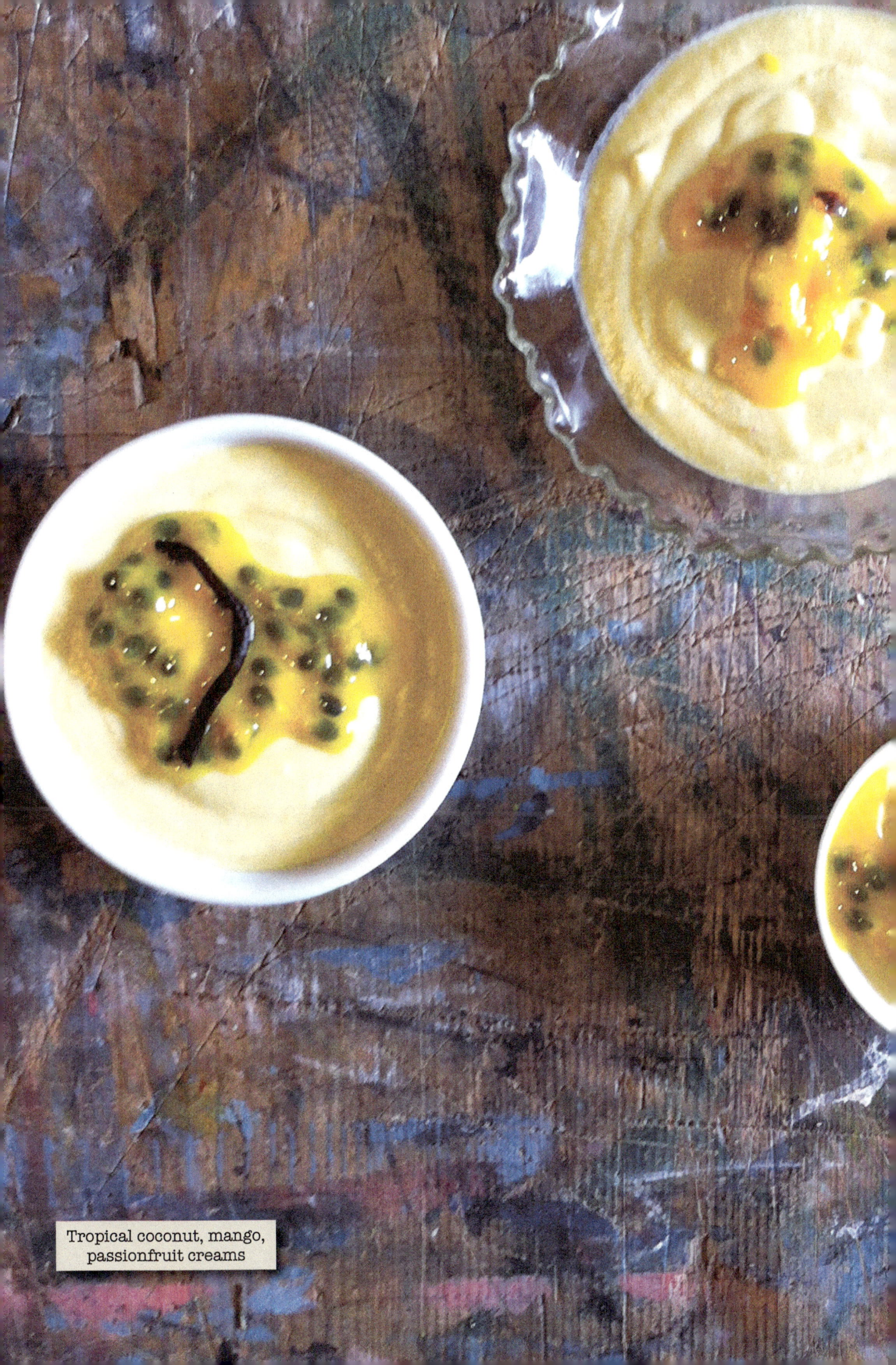

Blueberry jelly and gummies

Jelly is our treat, our first thing in the morning, our afternoon snack.

Its fun consistency is hard to beat when it comes to our children and they love to be able to join me when it comes to making it.

As I've already mentioned, a really good quality gelatine goes a long way to soothe inflamed gut lining. We try to have it every day in one form or another.

Experiment with whatever fruit you have.

We have done watermelon, nectarine, peach, the list goes on and on.

When I want my children to try herbal remedies, I make them in jelly form.

Lemon verbena leaves from the garden, finely grated ginger and lemon juice make a great jelly for tummy upsets like diarrhoea and nausea. Add raw honey to taste.

Fresh mint is lovely if you are looking for a mint jelly to go with your roast lamb.

Try using gelatine to make your cranberry sauce to go with your turkey this Christmas. Some people use sour cherries too.

Just whizz up the fruit in a blender or food processor and double the content by adding the same amount of filtered water.

I then get 2 tbs of boiling water and add 2.5 tsps of dissolved gelatine to every cup of fruit juice mixture I have.

If making gummies or jubes you need much more gelatine. I use 1½ tbs of gelatine dissolved in a little hot water for every ⅓ of a cup of freshly pressed fruit juice. Sweeten with honey if desired, a squeeze of lemon is also nice. A few drops of water kefir in the mix is also beneficial. Pour into silicon moulds and leave to set in the fridge.

Be sure to whisk the gelatine through quickly as it has a tendency to clump.

Then add the gelatine mixture to the rest of your fruit juice and give it one final stir.

Refrigerate until firm.

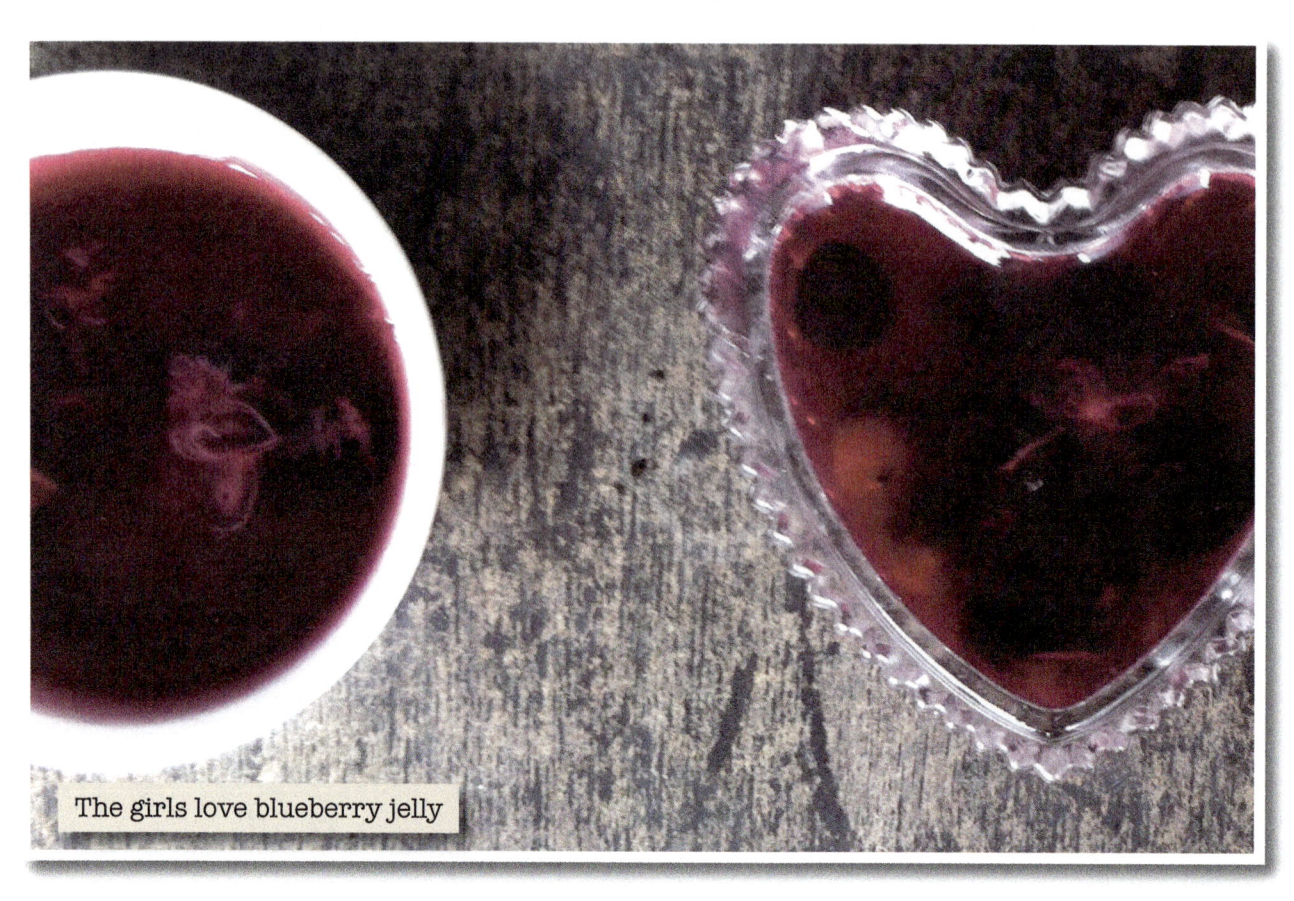

The girls love blueberry jelly

Drinks

Summer cocktails

Egyptian pink lemonade

A Summer fave that's pretty grown up but that the kids can have too.

Ingredients

- Hibiscus tea
- Orange blossom honey
- Lemon
- Mint leaves
- Mineral water.

Making it

1. Make a tea to the strength of your liking (I buy Hibiscus online on iherb).
2. Allow to cool and put into a pitcher with a cup of ice cubes. Add mineral water.
3. Sweeten with raw honey to taste and a squeeze of lemon.
4. Top with mint leaves.

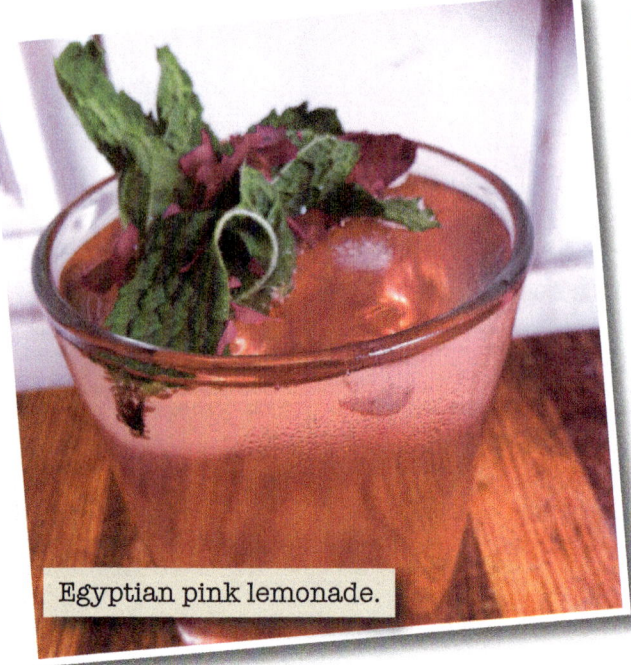

A healthy cocktail: Apple cider vinegar, mineral water, raw honey.

Ingredients

- 1 cap full of apple cider vinegar (I use one with the mother)
- 1 glass of mineral water
- 1 tsp of raw honey

Extra tip

This is a beautiful, festive drink for the non-drinker. Not only is it refreshing and delicious but apple cider vinegar has some massive claims to health fame.

From helping digestion and easing mozzie bite stings to fighting colds and arthritis, apple cider vinegar holds the title of one of nature's heavy weight medicines.

If you are going to take apple cider vinegar for health purposes you need to get a raw one with the "mother".

I have a cap full of it diluted in filtered water first thing on an empty stomach.

I then have it a couple of times a day and turn it into an evening cocktail if I'm not drinking.

Today we tried it with lemon verbena leaves we had growing in the garden and some ginger honey.

We then tried one with lemon thyme and orange blossom honey.

It's also lovely with just raw honey and a squeeze of lemon but you could add mint leaves, pomegranate jewels, little pieces of mango...

Have fun experimenting.

Egyptian pink lemonade.

Healthy cocktail

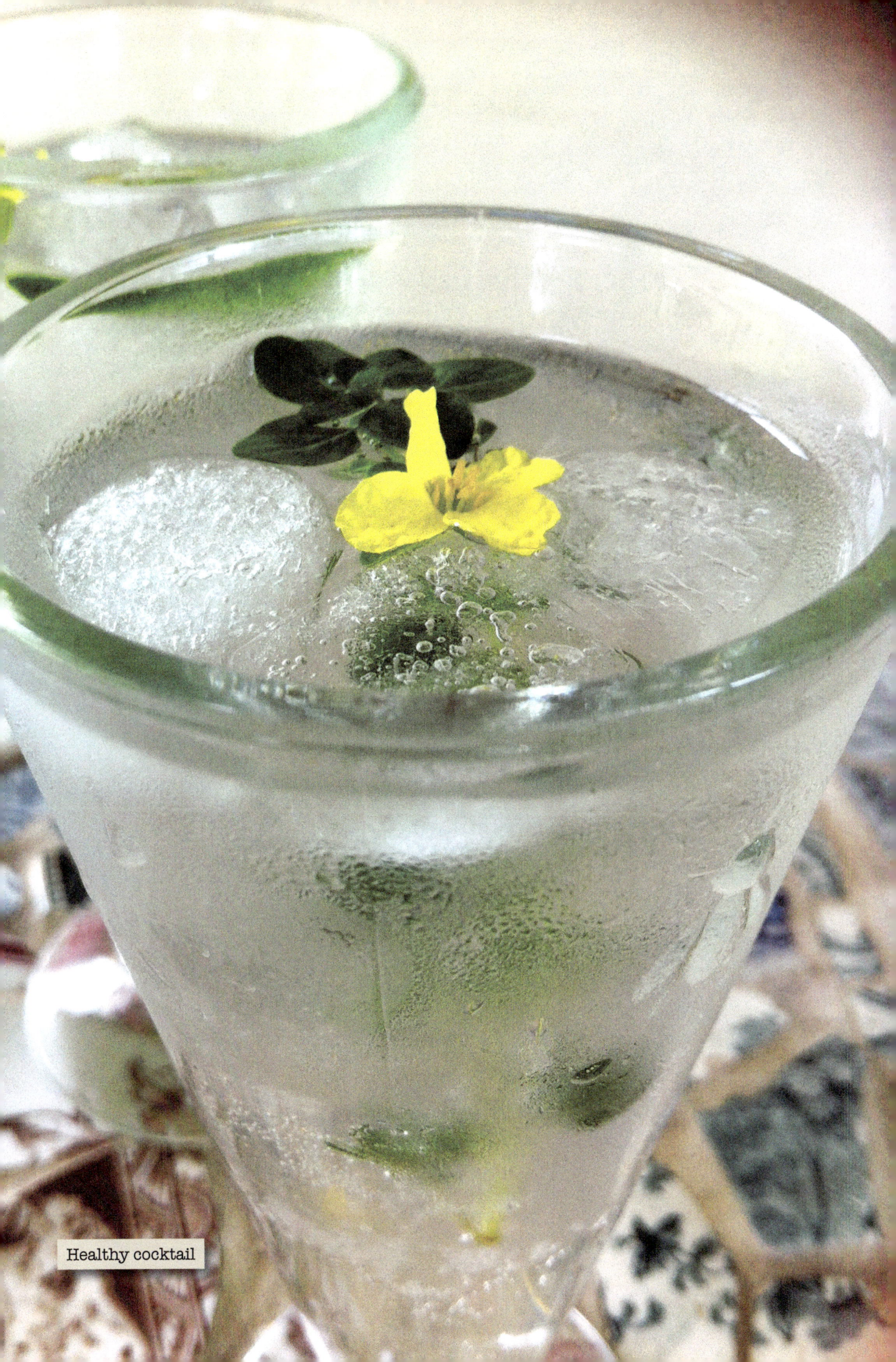

Beetroot kvass: A deeply cleansing tonic.

Beets are great for the liver. They help with constipation and in Chinese Medicine, they are said to be good for the blood.

Making it

1. Lacto-ferment them to make a lovely refreshing drink which many children love by getting a couple of organic beetroots, dice, and add 1 tsp of very good sea salt to every cup of filtered water to a medium-sized, sterilised jar with an air tight lid (about 750ml).
2. Leave for about 10 days on your kitchen bench top away from direct sunlight. Ferment time will vary depending on warmth of kitchen and time of year.
3. Strain off the liquid and put it in the fridge for a few more days.
4. When you taste the kvass from the fridge it should have a slight sour/sweet fizz to it. Dilute with water if too salty.

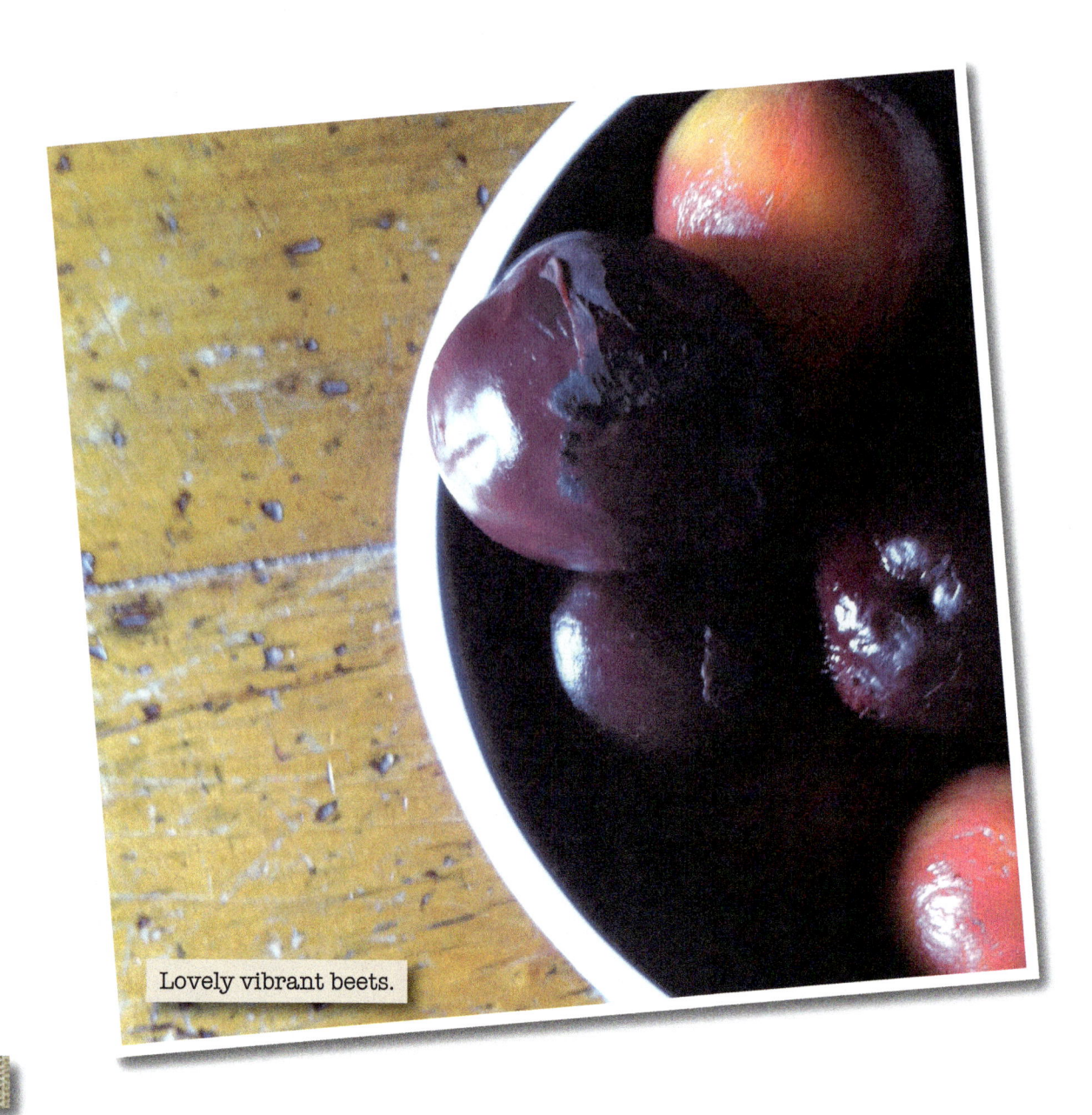

Lovely vibrant beets.

Beetroot Kavass.

Watermelon, young coconut, lemon & lime frappe

These were made on a beautiful summer's day. Cool breeze, warm low-tide sand pools to splash around in.

This is a great post-swim drink when you can still feel the salt on your skin.

The watermelon is a hit with most children and the coconut water is a great electrolyte. Be careful to choose a product that you trust if you are buying a packaged water.

The only way you can really be sure is to crack a young green coconut yourself.

> We made a double batch today and froze half to make some lovely little icy poles for this afternoon.

For a cocktail party, try adding some vodka to the mix. Pour into a long flat container and freeze. Take out about 45 minutes before serving and scrape with a fork. Serve them in martini glasses as a granita.

Ingredients
- 2 cups watermelon
- 1 cup coconut water
- Juice of one lemon and half a lime
- 1 cup of ice

Making it
This is super easy - adjust to your taste and leave out coconut and lemon if you wish. It would be fine with just ice or water.

1. Whiz up in a high speed blender and serve immediately.

Adult option
Add a ½ cup of vodka. If doing a cocktail.

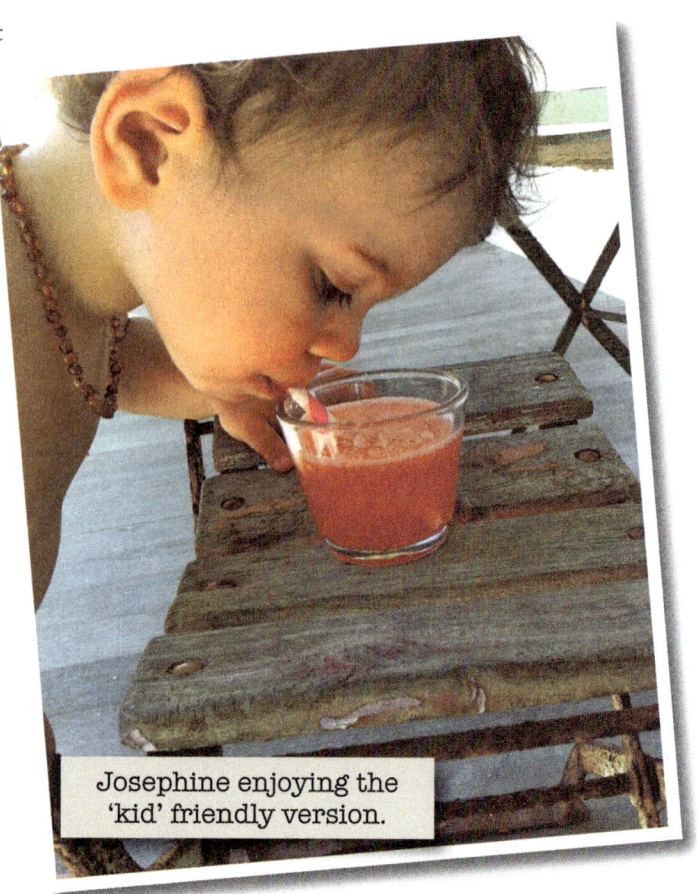

Josephine enjoying the 'kid' friendly version.

Watermelon, young coconut, lemon & lime frappe.

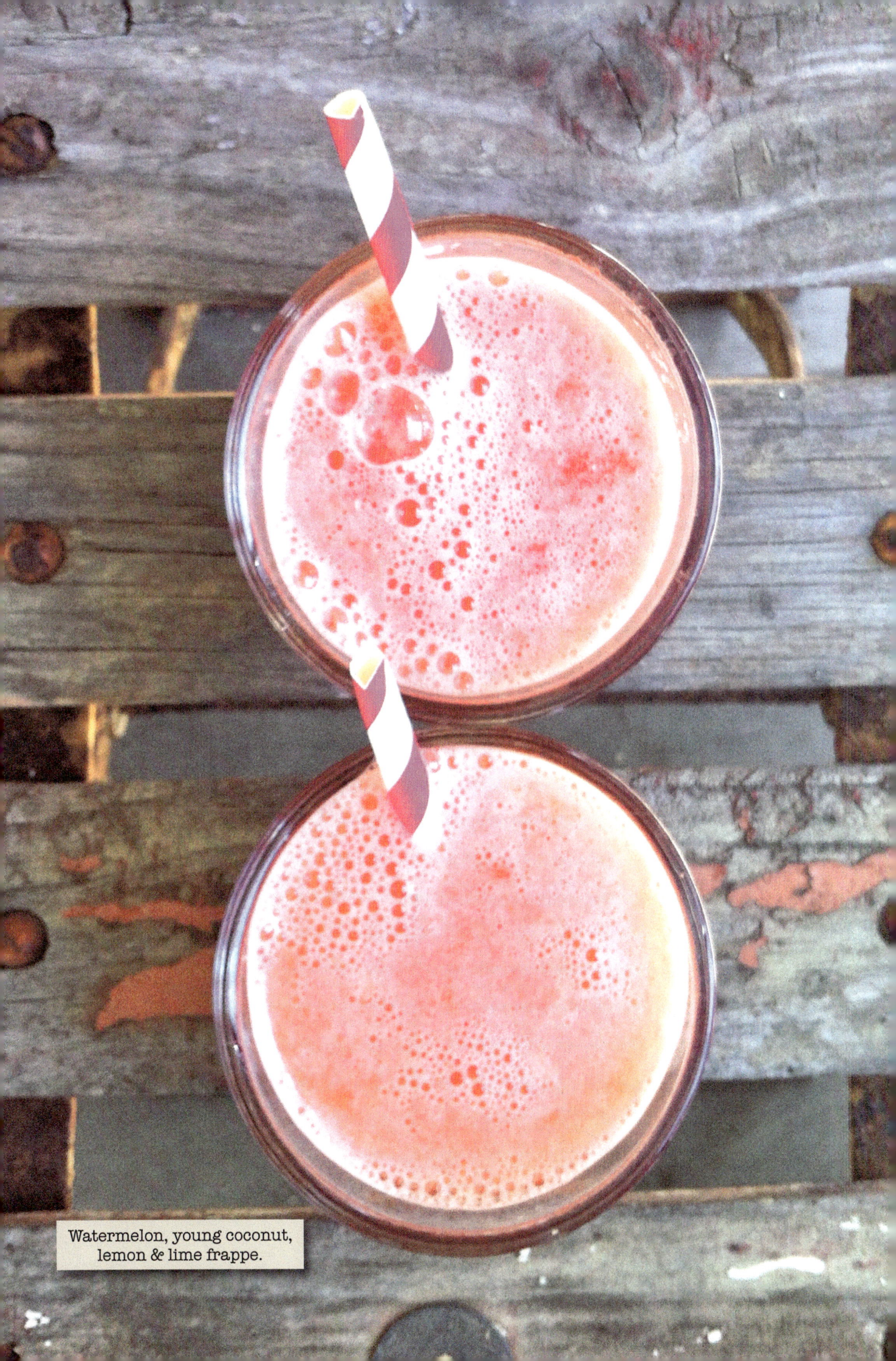

Green smoothies Vs Pink smoothies: Which one is right for you?

Everywhere I look I see green smoothies. They seem to be so many people's early morning go-to these days.

Kale, beet tops, silverbeet, mint, parsley – it's open slather on your veggie patch. I love the idea of getting all that nutrition into a delicious, power-packed, super quick liquid meal.

It's a no-brainer for someone who has great gut health, however, in our situation, where gut health is compromised, it's always a case of proceeding with caution.

Donna Gates who founded the Body Ecology Diet is right into the green smoothie. (http://bodyecology.com/recipes/market-green-smoothie.php)

She believes that keeping the vegetables in their whole, uncooked form whizzed up in a blender with just a little bit of green apple to slightly sweeten the deal is a way of helping you keep candida under control while helping you to clean and detoxify your liver – which is often one of the reasons why the gut gets into trouble.

UK-based neurologist and nutritionist Dr Natasha Campbell McBride - the creator of GAPS (Gut And Psychology Syndrome) - is more inclined to go for the traditional juicing option (www.gaps.me).

She believes in starting with just a teaspoon of carrot juice (or any other well-tolerated vegetable juice) and slowly increasing its amounts per day. According to Dr Campbell-McBride this slow introduction of juices will help to control any die-off or detox reactions a person may have.

Once you are tolerating a single vegetable juice (such as carrot juice), she recommends adding gradually other vegetables and fruit such as celery, lettuce, apple, greens and small amounts of beetroot. As the gut is more able to tolerate a variety of juiced vegetables, she recommends adding more fruit to make the juice more palatable.

Once the juices are fully introduced she recommends to start turning them into so-called GAPS Milkshakes, which are very nourishing and a great liver cleanser. To make GAPS milkshake for every glass of juice add one raw egg and 1-2 tablespoons of homemade sour cream (or coconut oil) to the juice and whisk.

Dietician Marieke Rodenstein of The Nutrition Practice (www.thenutritionpractice.com.au) says that raw fruit and veg (including raw fruit and veg smoothies and juices) can be particularly problematic for individuals who experience diarrhoea or loose stools.

"Raw food can promote or exacerbate these conditions," she says.

"Juicing, however, can be very beneficial for individuals who suffer from constipation. Green juices/smoothies can be problematic for some people, particularly if you have gut issues or an inflammatory condition."

Leafy greens contain oxalates, she explains, which are naturally occurring chemicals found in many plants, nuts and seeds.

Intestinal bacteria usually break down oxalates so that they can be eliminated via the faeces. If, however, you have gut dysbiosis or leaky gut, oxalates can enter into your bloodstream where they can interfere with nutrient absorption, impair enzymes and cause inflammation.

> "A common mistake that people make when preparing and consuming green smoothies or vegetable juices is failing to add some fat," she says.

"Many of the nutrients in vegetables are fat-soluble so you need to consume some fat with your juice/veg smoothie in order to absorb these nutrients," she says.

"Studies, like this one http://ajcn.nutrition.org/content/80/2/396.full, for example, have shown that individuals who consume salads with low-fat or non-fat dressings absorb far fewer nutrients from the vegetables than individuals who consume their salads with a higher fat dressing."

In our case, we started slowly with just a tiny bit of carrot juice, now, six months on, my little girl can tolerate a whole cup of juice first thing in the morning.

I make sure to add a bit of avocado and some cultured cream to the mix. If I have it on the go, I add beetroot kvass – another super easy probiotic drink. Enjoy.

Smoothies

Green smoothie
- 2 sticks of celery, blended
- Handful of mint leaves, blended
- ½ green apple, blended

You can add anything else to this base. People use beetroot tops, silverbeet, etc

(If you want to add fat, ½ an avocado will do it as would some cultured cream.)

Pink smoothie
- 1 stick of celery, juiced
- 1 carrot, juiced
- 1 green apple, juiced
- 2 tbs beetroot kvass
- 1 tbs cultured cream

(The more kvass and cream you use, the more pink it will go)

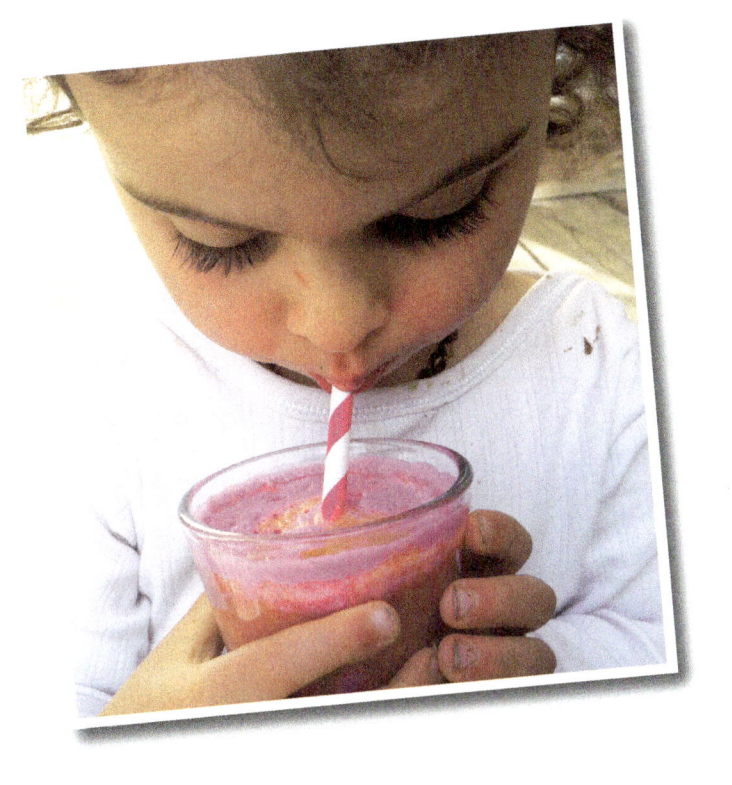

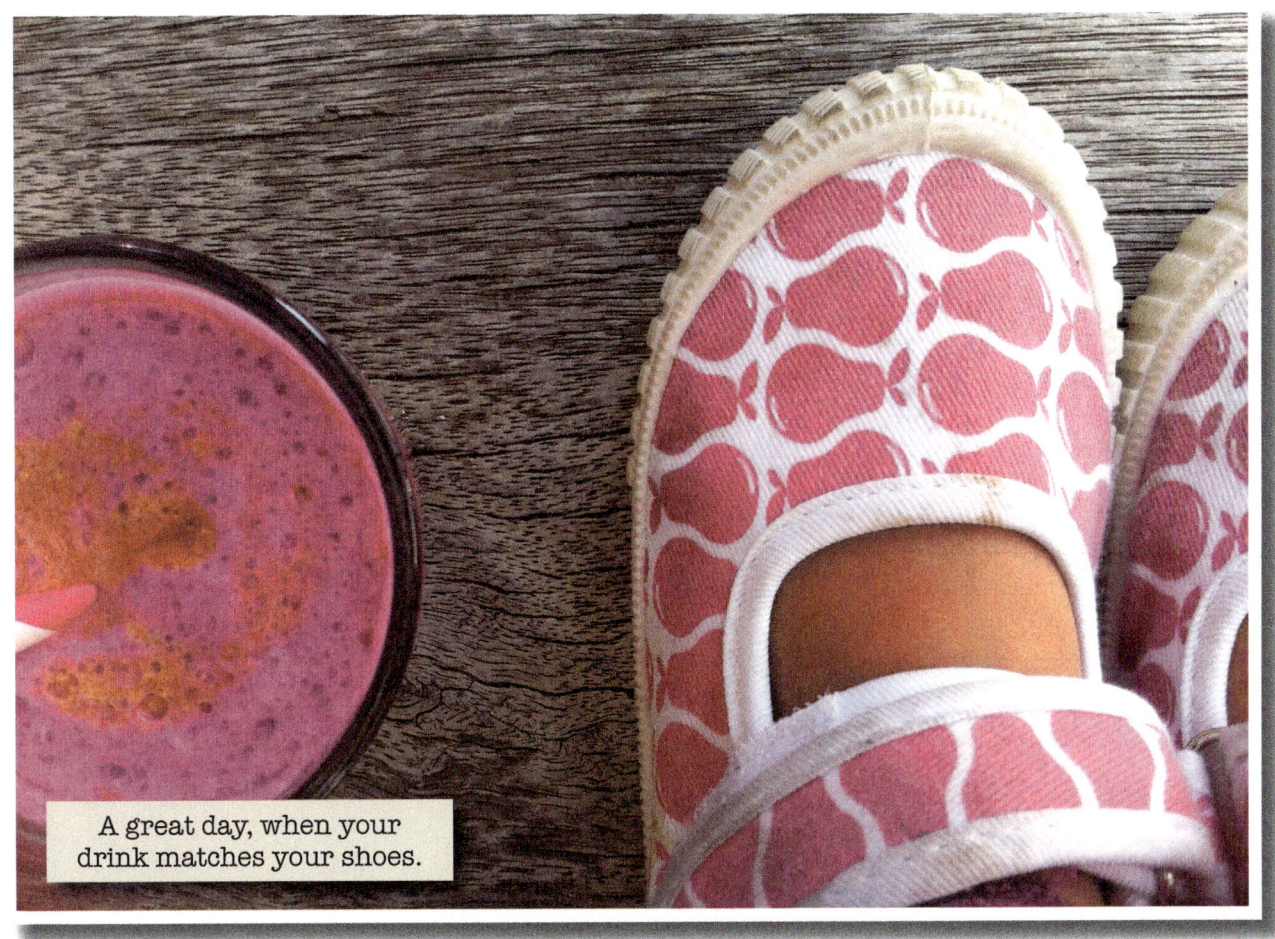

A great day, when your drink matches your shoes.

The real deal: Probiotic mango avocado lassi.

One sip and we were transported back to India. Sweet, tart and super refreshing.

Making lassi is all about using the whey from your home made yoghurt.

Whey is a beautiful thing.

It's full of good bacteria, great as a stand alone health tonic, a natural digestive (a must in all traditional Indian meals) and is a very cheap alternative to using a packet culture starter when making lacto-fermented foods.

When lacto-fermenting veggies you can get away with using just good quality salt, but if you are culturing fruit this summer, you really need a culture starter or whey.

Ingredients

- 2 cheeks of a large, ripe mango
- ¼ avocado
- 2 cups of whey, yoghurt or milk kefir

Making it

1. Whizz up with a stick blender and drink straight away.

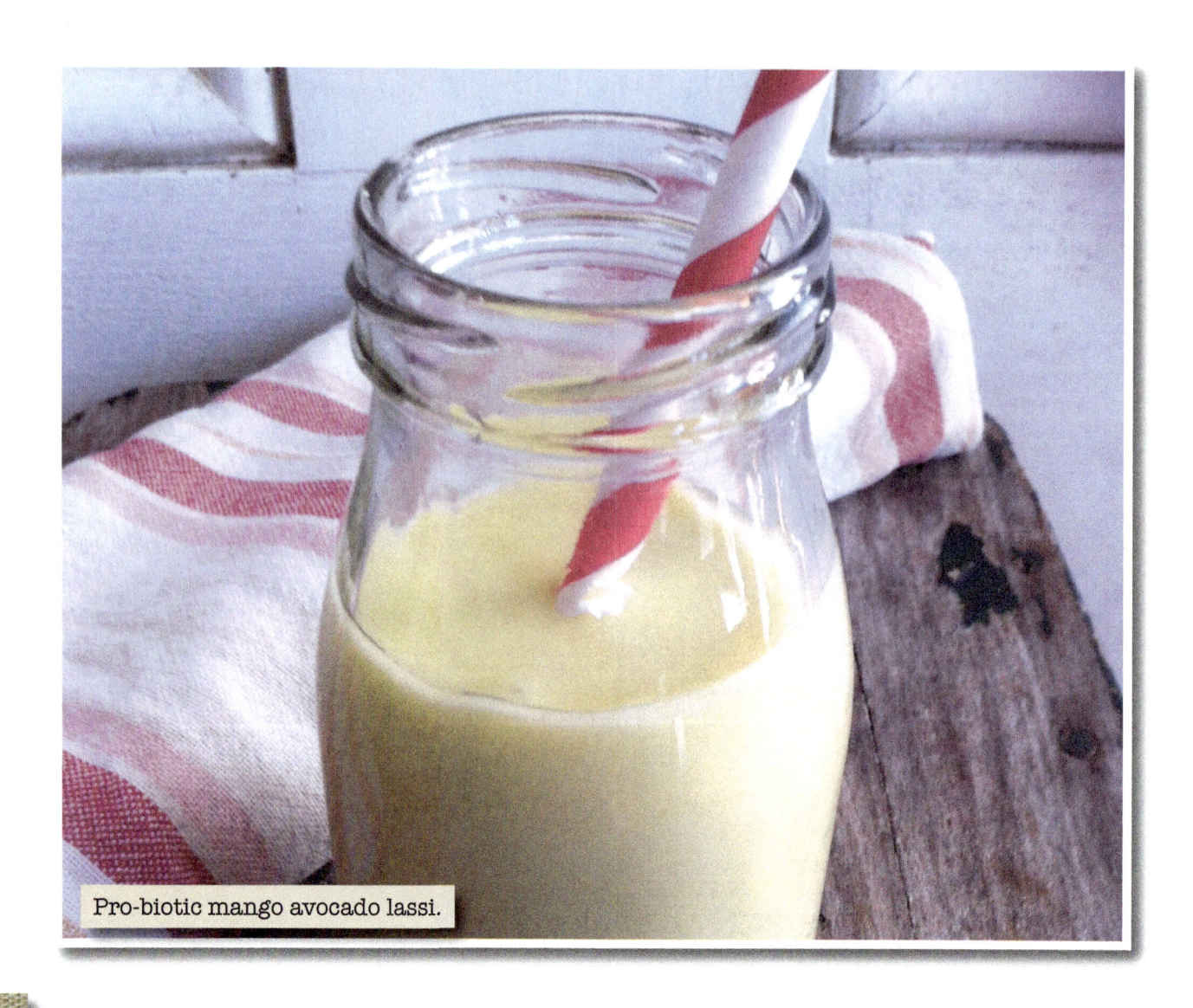

Pro-biotic mango avocado lassi.

For our friends with severe allergies.

When we first found out about Stevie's allergies, I was lost in the kitchen. It takes time but there are so many substitutes that the whole family can enjoy.

For parents whose children are attending kinder or school with allergic children, I thank you from the bottom of my heart for your part in helping these children remain safe.

I remember my time working as a news reporter for Australian Associated Press. I was attending the inquest of a little boy called Hamidur Rahman. In short, it was a long time ago. No-one was really aware of how deadly just a touch of an allergen or a spoonful of allergen could be. Essentially, this little boy was on school camp in a country location. He was dared to eat a spoonful of peanut butter. Knowing he was allergic, he took the dare but discretely ran to the toilet, where the peanut butter was found spat out in the sink. Within minutes, little Hamidur went into anaphylactic shock and died in his teacher's arms before an ambulance could arrive.

I never forgot this story. The devastated parents, the teacher who years on, was still a crying, ruined man, the coroner who so sensitively tried to reassure him that times were different then - there was nothing he could have done. The hardened journalists from all news outlets that cried with me as we wrote down every word.

This was the story that flashed through my mind when we were first handed our epipens. I burst out crying looking at our beautiful little 11-month-old little girl. I thought of little Hamidur.

We were told to avoid all allergens and traces of them until further notice.

My days of cooking from scratch had begun.

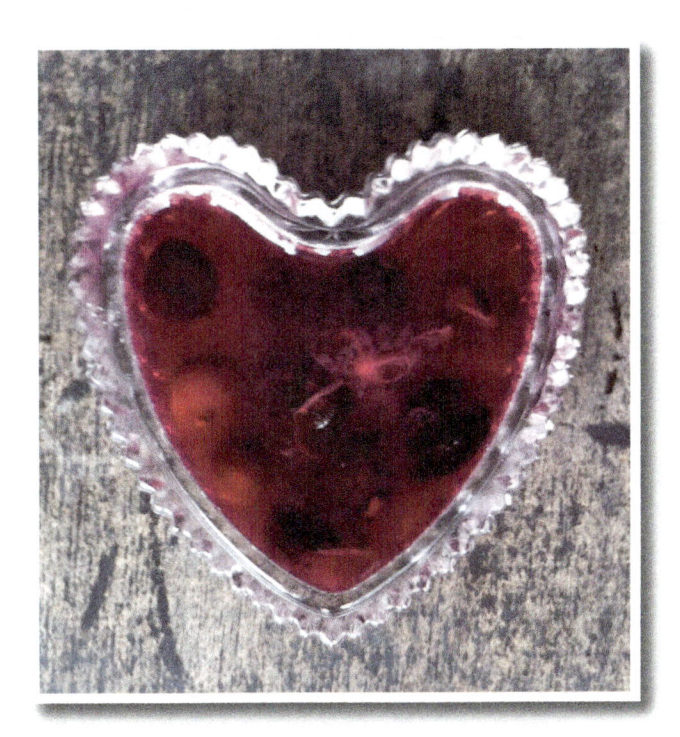

My lesson: No-body wants to see a child die. No-one would ever want to pack the sandwich or the food that killed a little boy or girl at school.

My task: Provide recipes, ideas and alternatives for all parents to help children be able to join in and stay safe.

There are known allergens included in this book, however, many ingredients are very easily substituted.

Please be mindful to be nut free when using these recipes for kinder or school.

Afterword

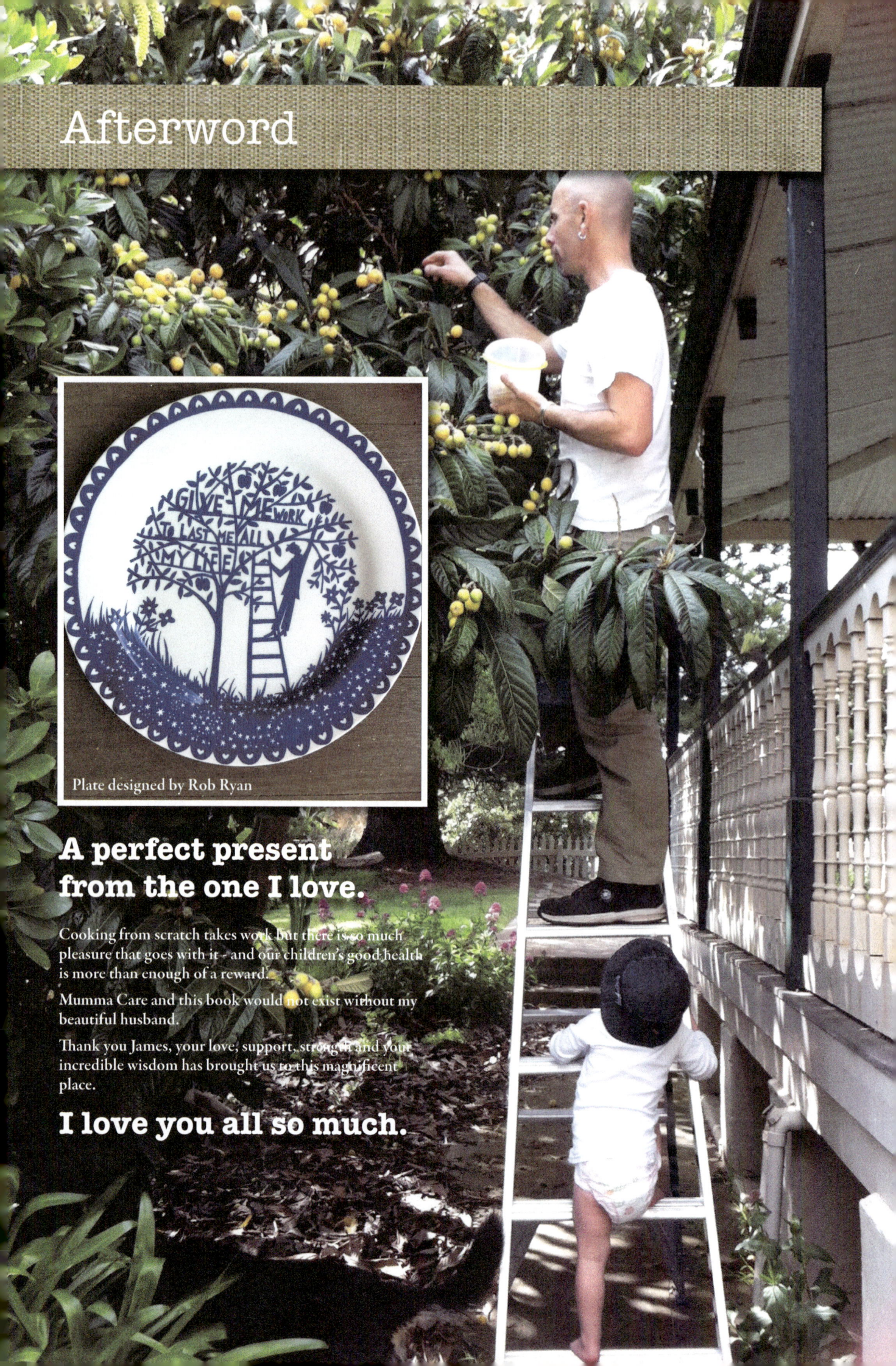

Plate designed by Rob Ryan

A perfect present from the one I love.

Cooking from scratch takes work but there is so much pleasure that goes with it - and our children's good health is more than enough of a reward.

Mumma Care and this book would not exist without my beautiful husband.

Thank you James, your love, support, strength and your incredible wisdom has brought us to this magnificent place.

I love you all so much.

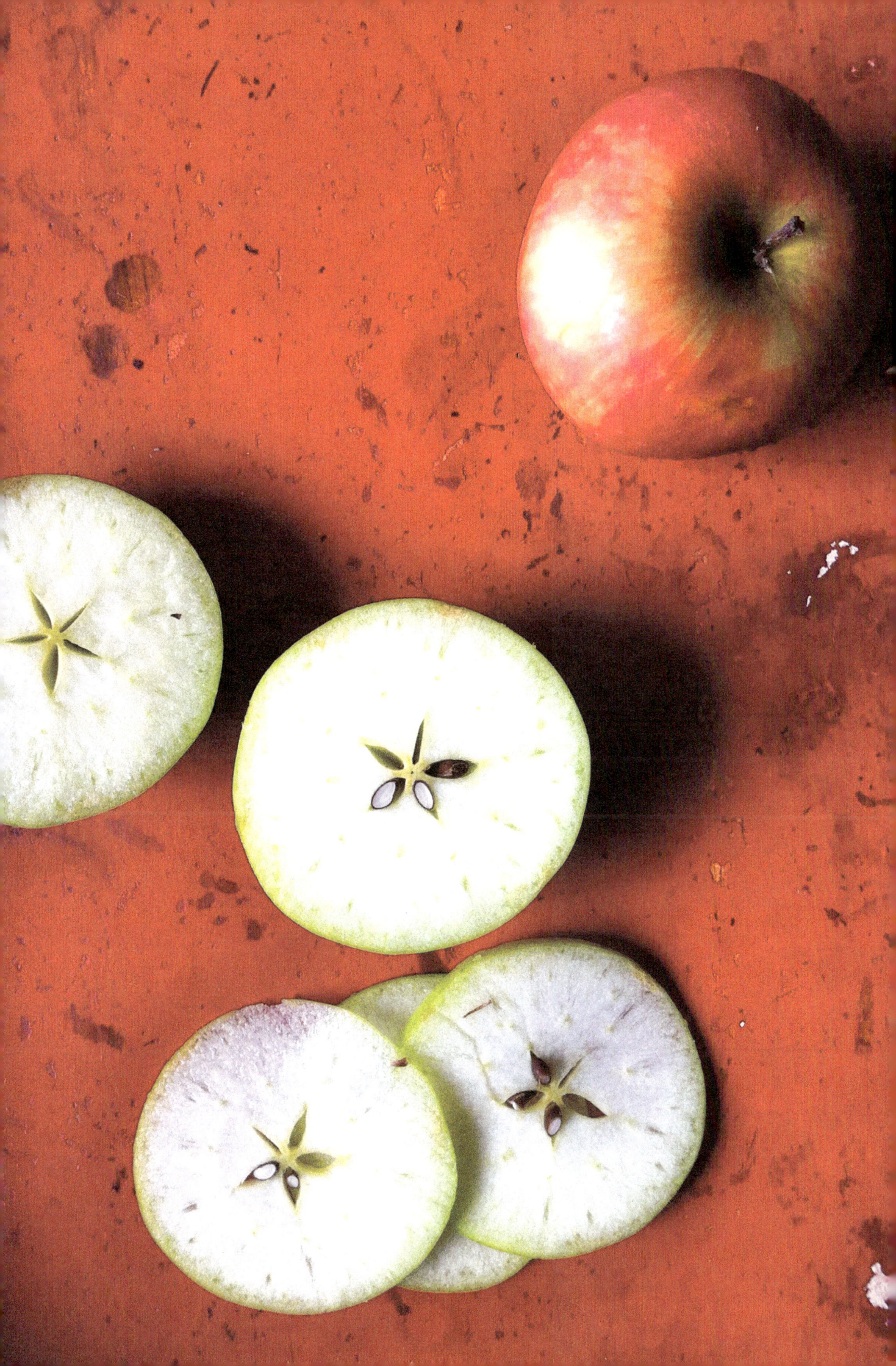

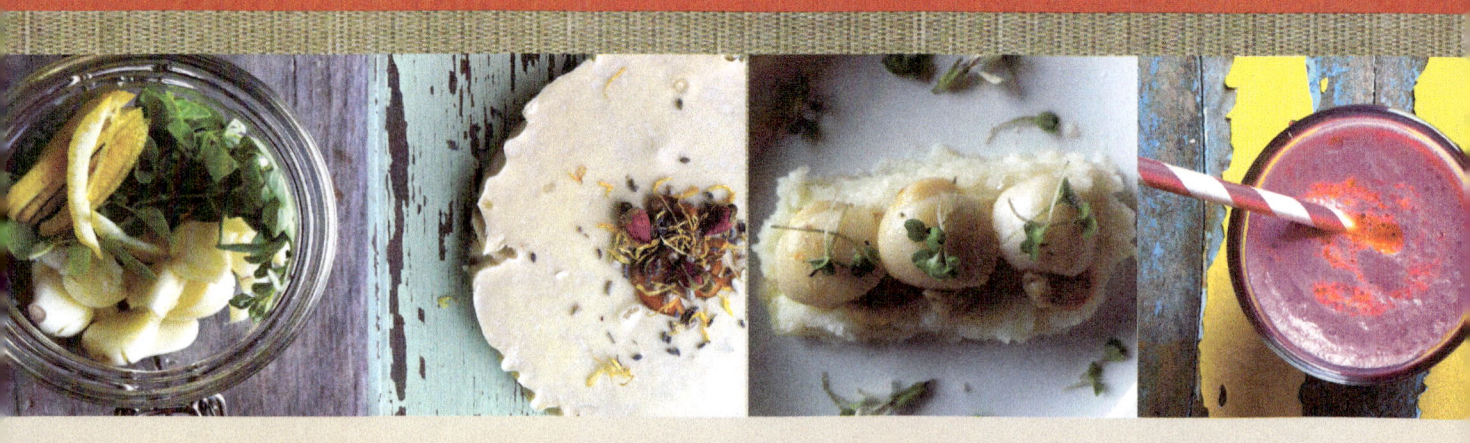

"Dear Nicole, Thank you very much for your email and the book! Stories such as yours are so heart-warming and inspiring! I love your book, the recipes are simple and easy to follow and the photos are beautiful."

Neurologist, nutritionist and author of the GAPS Diet, Natasha Campbell-McBride

"How beautiful and inspiring this book is! Congratulations Nicole on sharing your story that enables others to transform food into medicine. Your book is captivating as each word emanates the love that you have for food and for your children.

As a mother, I have thoroughly enjoyed turning each page of this book. I feel inspired to further optimize my family's diet and boost my son's love of food. The colours and the flavours of the foods that you combine together fill my heart (and my stomach) with excitement. I can't wait to bring this nourishing food to our family's table!

As a doctor, I am grateful to have this as a resource to recommend to any of my patients who suffer from allergies, chronic conditions or keen to improve their health! A large number of my patients have undergone phenomenal healing after taking steps to improve their diet and heal their gut. How happy I am to have your book that simply explains how best to do this and explores with the readers how food really is the best medicine. Thank you!"

Dr Fiona Enkelmann
MBBS FRACGP MPH

"Guided by the principle of 'let your food be your medicine' Nicole's experience of transforming her daughters' health through diet is a testament to the many ways that food can heal the body.

Achieving better health is within reach for each and everyone of us and The Alchemy Cookbook is a wonderful companion to get you back in your kitchen and cooking your way to a healthier you.

Not only are Nicole's recipes, which she has so beautifully photographed, nutrient dense and delicious, they are also practical, easy and enjoyable to make.

This wonderful book will inspire you to believe in the power to heal your body, one recipe at a time. I can't recommend it highly enough."

Dietitian and Nutritionist Marieke Rodenstein.
GAPS Practitioner and MINDD certified

"Hi nic, thanks for sharing your book. it looks great! keep fermenting and sharing your fermentation fervour."

Author of Wild Fermentation and fermentation expert Sandor Katz